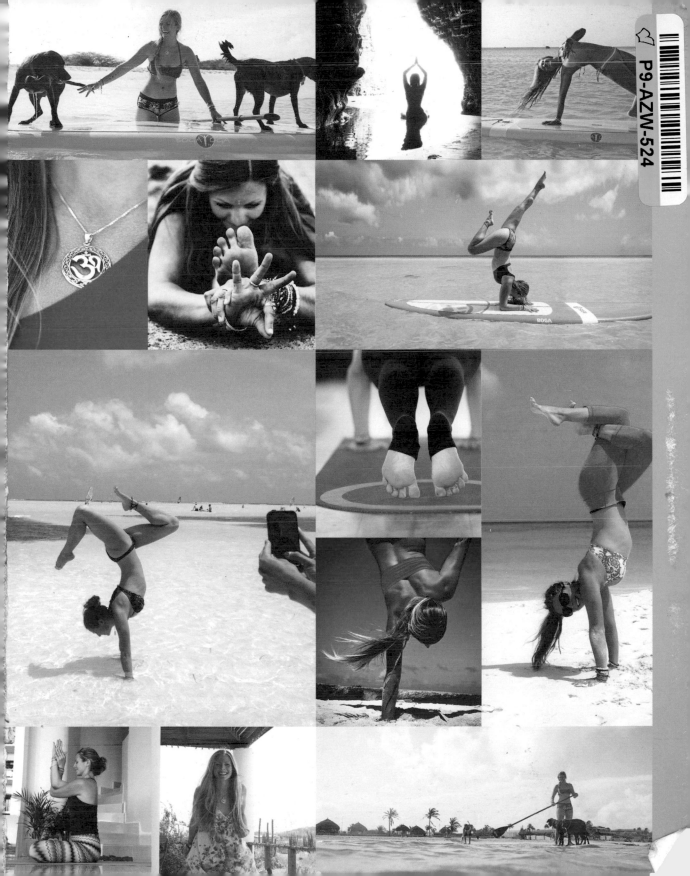

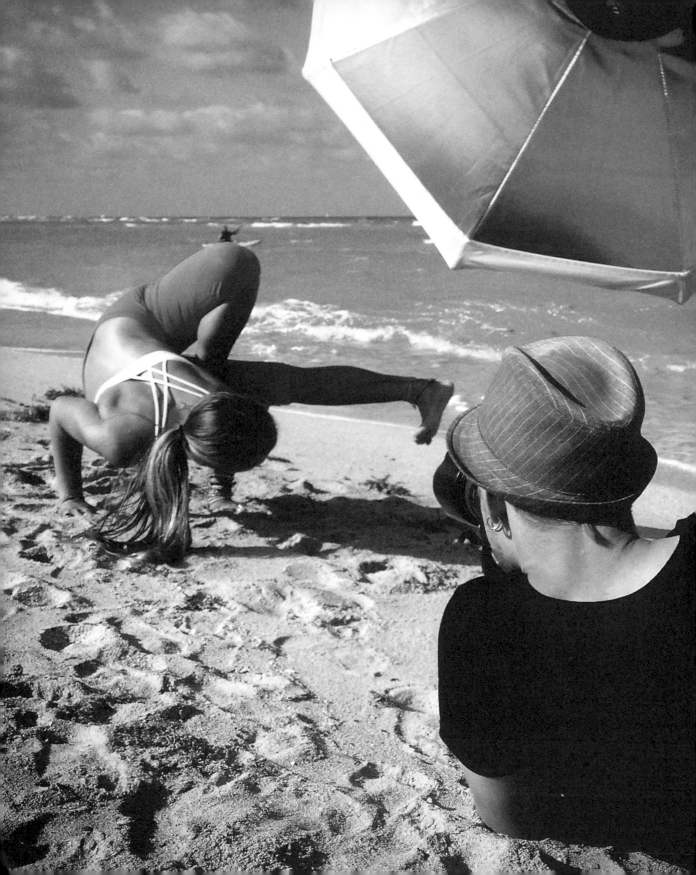

RACHEL BRATHEN

Yoga Girl

TOUCHSTONE

New York   London   Toronto   Sydney   New Delhi

Touchstone
An Imprint of Simon & Schuster, Inc.
1230 Avenue of the Americas
New York, NY 10020

This publication contains the opinions and ideas of its author. It is intended
to provide helpful and informative material on the subjects addressed
in the publication. It is sold with the understanding that the author and
publisher are not engaged in rendering medical, health, or any other kind
of personal professional services in the book. The reader should consult his
or her medical, health, or other competent professional before adopting
any of the suggestions in this book or drawing inferences from it.
The author and publisher specifically disclaim all responsibility for any liability,
loss or risk, personal or otherwise, which is incurred as a consequence, directly
or indirectly, of the use and application of any of the contents of this book.

First Touchstone trade paperback edition March 2015

TOUCHSTONE and colophon are registered
trademarks of Simon & Schuster, Inc.

For information about special discounts for bulk purchases,
please contact Simon & Schuster Special Sales at
1-866-506-1949 or business@simonandschuster.com.

The Simon & Schuster Speakers Bureau can bring authors
to your live event. For more information or to book an event
contact the Simon & Schuster Speakers Bureau at 866-248-3049
or visit our website at www.simonspeakers.com.

Manufactured in the United States of America

1   3   5   7   9   10   8   6   4   2

Library of Congress Cataloging-in-Publication Data
Brathen, Rachel.
Yoga girl / Rachel Brathen.
pages   cm
Originally published in 2014 in Sweden by Bonnier Fakta.
1. Brathen, Rachel.   2. Yoga teachers—Sweden—Biography.
3. Yoga teachers—Aruba—Biography.   I. Title.
RA781.67.B72 2015
613.7'046092—dc23
[B]   2014047319

ISBN 978-1-5011-0676-7
ISBN 978-1-5011-0677-4 (ebook)

For every single person who's ever stepped on a yoga mat.
And for those out there who haven't . . . especially for you.

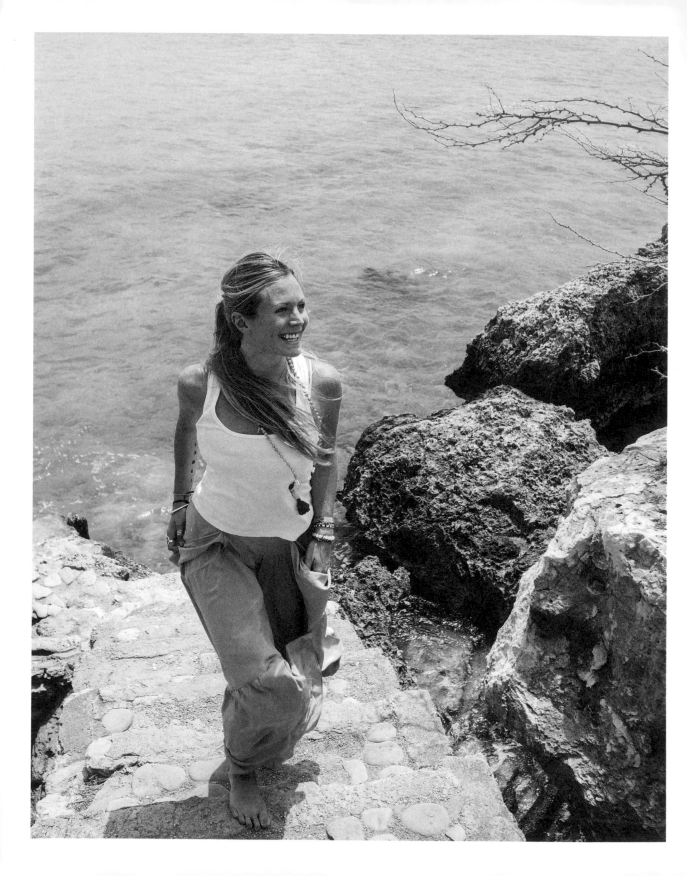

Contents

INTRODUCTION _____ I

CHAPTER 1
Yoga Every Damn Day _____ 2

CHAPTER 2
To love what is ahead, you must
love what has come before _____ 20

CHAPTER 3
Not all those who wander are lost _____ 46

CHAPTER 4
The body is a place
for the soul to reside in _____ 74

CHAPTER 5
Going with the flow _____ 100

CHAPTER 6
Love over fear _____ 118

CHAPTER 7
Moments of silence _____ 140

ACKNOWLEDGMENTS _____ 156

INDEX _____ 158

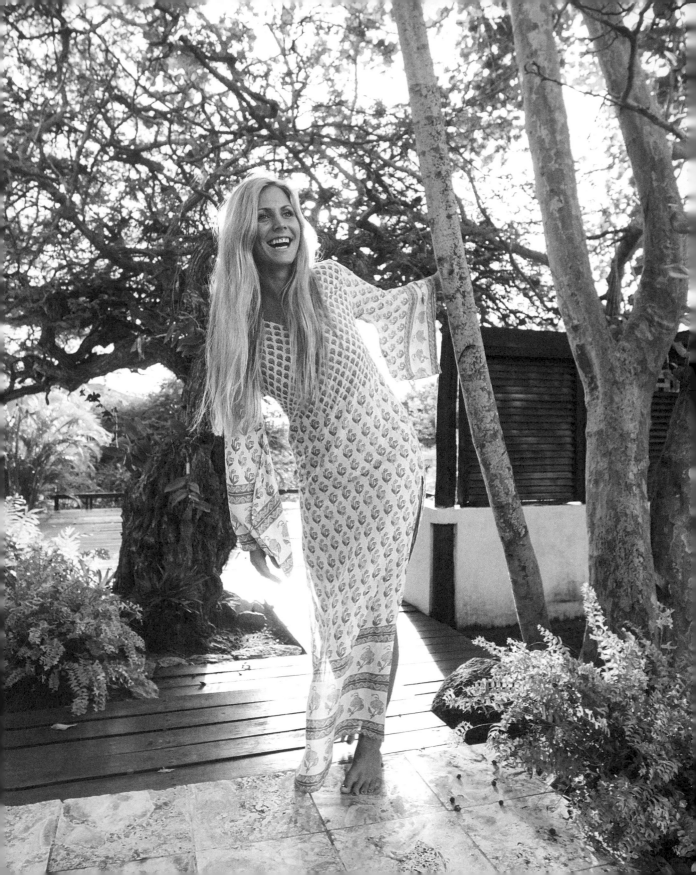

Yoga Girl

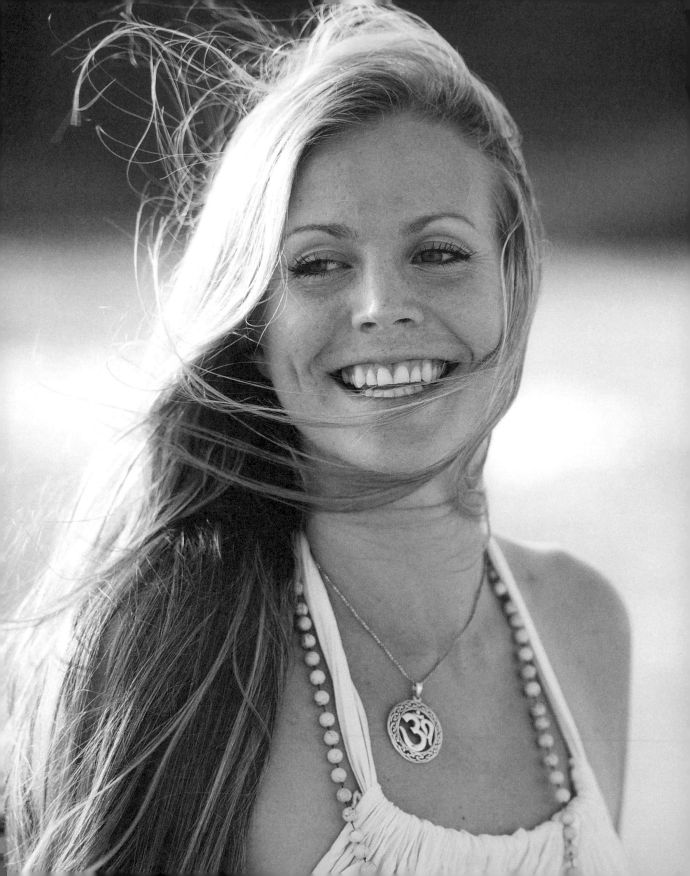

Introduction

Welcome to life as a yoga girl! Or yoga boy, for that matter. Yoga is a practice for anyone and everyone, and I'm here to share with you the big secret of finding success and balance in your life, yogi style.

The secret is, there is none. There is no grand recipe for a perfect life. In today's fast-paced society we often find ourselves looking for a quick fix, the next big thing to make us feel better, which is why we see new health trends and diets taking the world by storm every other week. I am not here to announce the newest weight-loss technique or to tell you that you should be eating fewer carbs or more carbs or no carbs (ah, that's it!) or whatever fad is hitting the Internet this morning. I am not here to tell you to change your life so that you can be better.

I'm here to tell you you are good enough the way you already are.

Shocking, I know. Even though we are a decade and a half into the twenty-first century, sending people to the moon on vacation and connecting through the virtual world in more ways than ever before, there is still a fundamental flaw in how we treat one another, and most of all, in how we treat ourselves. *We do not love ourselves enough.* We run around trying to find ways to change our bodies, our health, our love lives, our work—anything to make us feel whole and happy. But the faster we run, the faster we miss the point. We all search for balance, but finding this does not lie in the latest health trend. Balance comes from slowing down, from taking deep breaths, from understanding your body and what it needs. It comes from accepting who you are and loving yourself every step of the way.

For me, yoga was the way to get there. Although yoga is a practice that has been around for more than five thousand years, it's well adapted to the culture we live in and it's getting more popular every day. The world of yoga is so full of different styles, teachers, classes, online videos, and gadgets these days that it can be hard to navigate. My aim with this book is to give you an idea of what life as a yogi can entail, and to help you get back to the root of the practice: creating moments of silence. These moments are when the real breakthroughs happen, when we come back to our priorities, our focus, and the love we have for ourselves and the people around us. Yoga involves much more than physical poses practiced on a yoga mat. In fact, there are beautiful ways to use what we learn from this practice and bring it out into the world. I hope to inspire you to be the best you can be, and to accept and embrace every single aspect of what that means. 🌸

CHAPTER 1

Yoga Every Damn Day

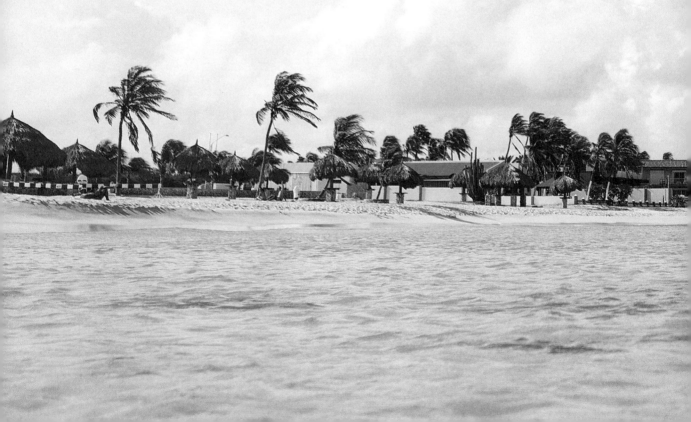

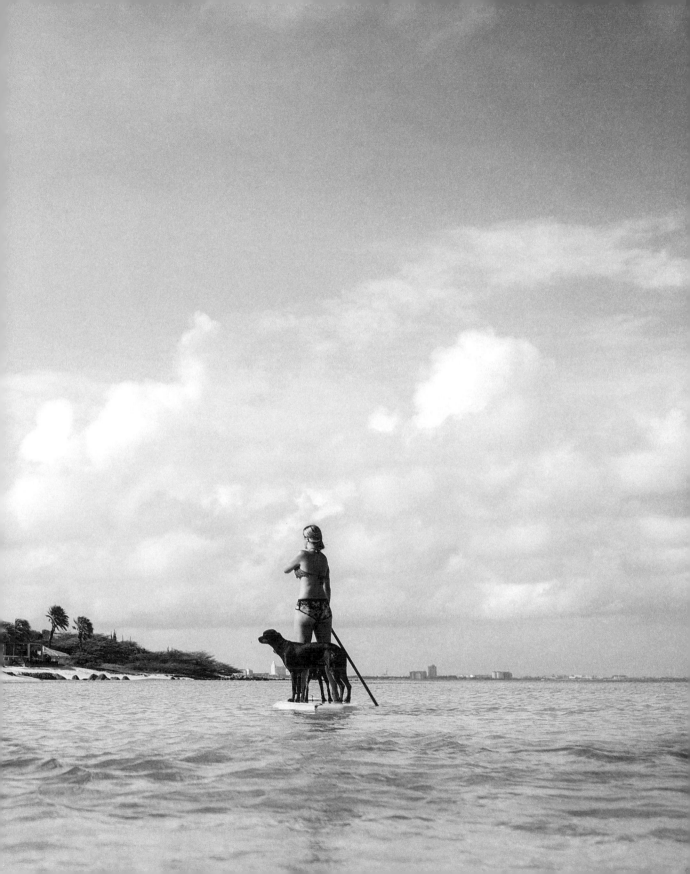

I firmly believe that real change and true happiness come from acceptance. Accepting our bodies, accepting who we are, and accepting the situation we are in. Many of the insecurities we struggle with daily come from thinking that things should be different from reality.

We live in a society that continuously harps on everything that we should change in our lives. We need to improve, do better, look better, feel better. We should lose weight, gain muscle, eat healthier, get better jobs, buy nicer clothes, get shinier hair, earn more money. Only rarely are we told that we are good enough just the way we are.

There is a big difference between genuinely wanting to change something about our way of life and feeling that we need to change because we have to alter who we are in order to be accepted and fit in. Where do you live on that spectrum? And what is it you are looking to change? If you are like most people, there are probably many things you'd like to see different in your life. My question is why. Throughout your life, who has told you that you are not good enough? Where did you get the idea? Most of the time the judgments we feel come from no one other than ourselves. No one judges you the way you do. When it comes to creating a happy, healthy life, we need to start from the right place. No matter what you want to change in your life—lose weight, de-stress, build a career—it needs to come from a place of genuine intention.

We can make changes in our lives based on love or on fear. Do you want to lose ten pounds because you know it would be good for your heart and you'd feel so much better? Or do you want to lose ten pounds so you'll fit into your skinny jeans and look better in a bikini? Maybe the answer is all of the above, but there is a very real difference between them. True, lasting, effortless change comes from taking action from a place of love. From the heart. Does your heart give a damn about what you look like in a bikini? I highly doubt that. However, it probably does cares about your ability to move freely, to be strong, and to feel healthy.

Caring for our well-being has to start from within, and this is also one of the most important foundations of the yoga practice. We need to direct our attention inward and connect to the breath. Focusing on our breath keeps us present, calms the mind, and allows us to develop the awareness of the body we need to practice with care and compassion. If we are not fully present, we are no longer practicing yoga but are simply doing exercises and stretches on a yoga mat. Cultivating this awareness begins with the

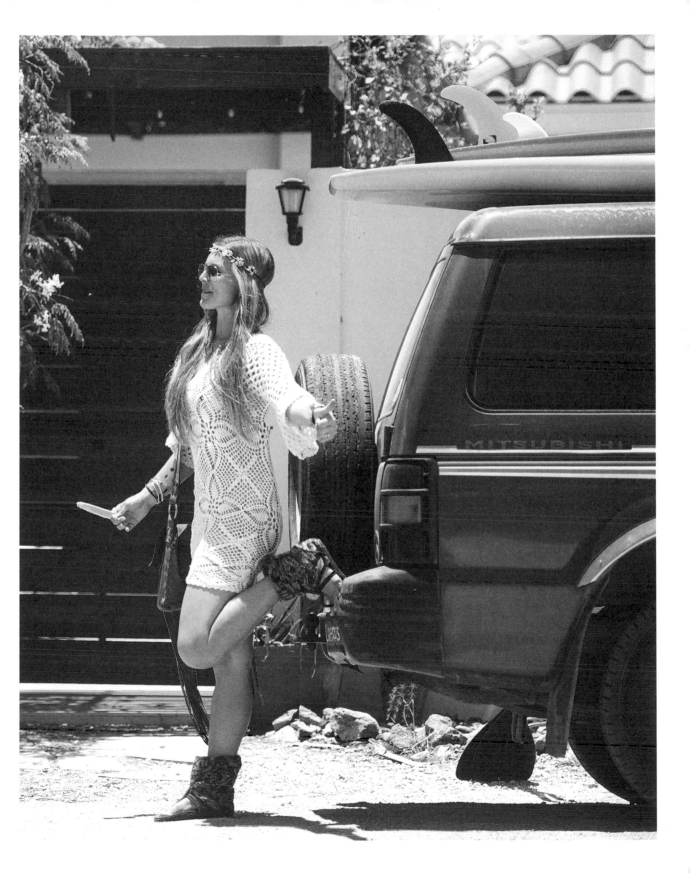

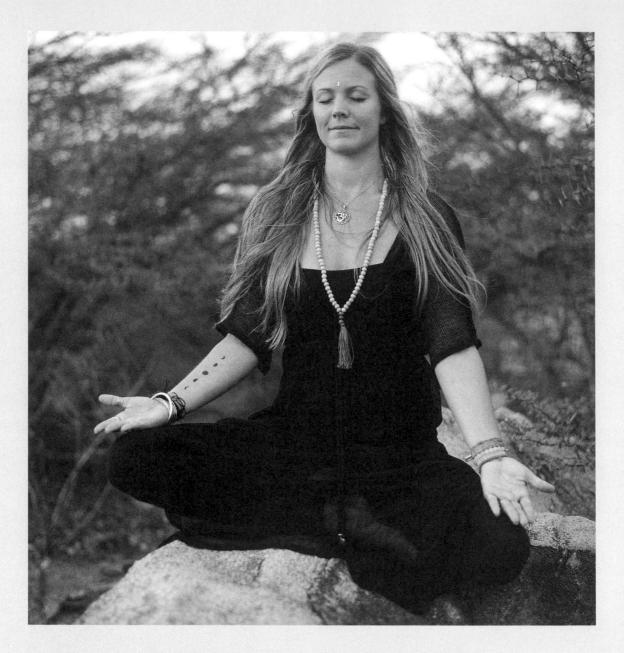

Take time either right before or right after your practice to sit in silence for a few moments. Set your intentions for the day, breathe deeply, and take a minute to extend gratitude to all of the beautiful things you have in your life. Bow your head to the earth. This is a small gesture of reverence and gratitude that helps us look within and direct our attention toward the happiness we have in life. After my practice I always drink a big green smoothie or a large green juice before heading out to embrace whatever life has in store for me that day.

> *"You don't need to change anything about
> who you are to start a yoga practice."*

───────────────

breath and is what eventually turns our chattering minds into quiet places for contemplation and acceptance.

This might sound complicated, but it's not. Actually, it's so simple our minds like to make it complex! Our minds do this, by the way. The ego likes to take what's simple and make it into a problem to solve so that it stays busy. A question I get all the time is "How could I ever become a yogi? I can't sit still!" or "I can't do yoga, I like to eat meat!"

If you believe practicing yoga means you need to get up at four every morning, eat only rice and vegetables, and spend most of the day sitting in the lotus position while humming "Om," think again. (However, if you practice long enough, you may find that sitting for a long time in lotus position can be quite rewarding. But you'll also learn that the poses practiced are not the be-all and end-all of why we do what we do.) As yogis, we simply strive for balance—in body, mind, and soul. Note the word *strive*, meaning that we continuously work and aim for balance. Balance is not something that shows up one day and is suddenly here to stay; it's the result of creating moments of mindfulness and gratitude throughout our day. That's why it's called a practice—it never ends.

You don't need to change anything about who you are to start a yoga practice. Adding yoga to your life does not mean you need to change everything about your daily life. You can be a yogi and still enjoy wine with dinner. You can practice yoga and work a corporate job. You can do yoga and forget to recycle when your day gets too busy. The definition of a real yogi is not someone who greets every person with a smile and a bow, but someone who goes with the flow of life and takes each moment as it comes. A real yogi has ups and downs just like anyone else. A real yogi does his or her best to greet each person with a smile, yes, but a real yogi also respects the roller coaster that is this life and allows emotions to arise when needed. Real yogis are simply those who live well, doing their best with what they have. On and off the yoga mat.

Balance is key in everything you do. So dance all night long and practice yoga the next day. Drink wine, but don't forget your green juice. Eat chocolate when your heart wants it and kale salad when your body needs it. Wear high heels on Saturday and walk barefoot on Sunday. Go shopping at the mall and then sit down and meditate in your bedroom. Live high and low. Move and stay still. Embrace all sides of who you

"Yoga creates space where we once were stuck."

are and live your authentic truth! Be brave and bold and spontaneous and loud, and let that complement your ability to find silence and patience and modesty and peace. Aim for balance. Make your own rules and don't let others tell you how to live according to theirs.

When you first begin, remember that we are all different, with different backgrounds, bodies, and circumstances. You must begin from where you are. Focus on what's going on in your own body and stay as mindful as you can while practicing. Be patient. The second your mind starts to interfere—*I should be doing better than this*; *The person next to me is much more flexible than I am*; *I'm not good enough* (all very common thoughts that come up in the beginning)—just keep bringing your focus back to the breath. Start where you are. Use what you have. Do what you can. Focus on the practice and try not to become hung up on the result.

With time, you'll notice changes within the body, the mind, and the breath. Yoga makes us strong but flexible. Yoga creates space where we once were stuck. Yoga cultivates a quiet mind and inspires concentration. Yoga allows the breath to grow deeper. Yoga is a space where, with practice, we can become more present in our day. And the deeper we go in our practice, the more natural it will be to take the yoga off the mat and into the rest of our lives.

The mind has a tendency to seek out worst-case scenarios. When we are immersed in thought, we often find ourselves stuck in repetitive thinking, judgment, labels, and negativity. The mind can be a great tool *when used correctly*. It's when the mind takes over and we can no longer control what goes on inside our heads that anxiety or regret arises. Moving our bodies with the breath and cultivating moments of deep presence are ways to quiet the mind, and this is exactly what yoga is. Movement. Breath. Uniting the body with the mind and creating a place of silence. When you live only in the mind, you will find yourself constantly reacting to what goes on around you, often with fear or worry. We all have had some negative experiences in our past, large or small, and to protect us from further pain, the mind does what it can to prevent them from happening again. Say you were once hurt or left by a loved one. The next time you meet someone you could fall in love with, you might find yourself reacting to or treating this person in a way that you might not have before. Always reacting to life means living from the past.

Yoga gives us the tools to greet each moment in life with the fresh eyes of the present moment. Just because a past love hurt you doesn't mean the next one will. And walking through life with our hands held out in front of us feeling for obstacles means we will miss out on much of the beauty of life. To love means to take risks. And there is love all around! If you meet new people with an open mind instead of with fear, you are likely to have quite a different experience with them.

For me this has been one of the greatest lessons I've learned from yoga: acting instead of reacting. Yoga has helped me create space between the situations that come at me; I don't have to react right away anymore. I can sit back, take it all in, and see the situation for what it is. There is much less drama in my life now than there has ever been. I used to confront people in order to start a fight or to create a big argument. Now I see confrontations as a way to come to an understanding and perhaps even correct the misperceptions we have about one another.

There is no need to change your habits to make space for a yoga practice. Start practicing yoga from where you are today, and let the practice change you. The more often you come to the mat, on your own or in a class, the easier it will be to make healthy decisions throughout the rest of your day. When you're listening more to your body, you'll find that it's not as difficult to eat well. With awareness of your body you'll find it easier to stay away from sugar or alcohol or whatever it is that you're looking to remove from your diet. Or perhaps you will realize that the foods you are eating are just fine, nothing to obsess over at all! The bottom line is, you will be more conscious about how your body feels and how sensitive it is to what you put in it. Maybe that second helping of food didn't make you feel better, after all. When we live more in the body and less in the mind, those choices that were so overwhelming before become easier to make. I know that when I really listen to my body, it very rarely wants two huge helpings of food. If I reach for more, it's probably because I'm busy talking and socializing or I'm feeling emotional. If I stay mindful, I'll be able to tell when I'm full. Much of what we eat in a day is simply a result of boredom! I'm not promising you'll stop wanting dessert or wine or all the good things that come with life (or every Friday night) just because you start practicing yoga. You'll simply be more receptive to what your body wants and needs. And this is the very first step to a healthy you.

As a yogi you will learn that you can have your cake and eat it, too; there is no need to feel guilty about your diet or your body. Life is about finding happiness. Balance. Love. Yoga is a beautiful tool to help you find all those things you've been looking for, and the time to start is right now.

How you wake up in the morning sets the tone for the rest of your day. If you've decided to make yoga a part of your daily life, why not start right away? Think about the first thing you usually do when you wake up. Do you check your e-mail? Drink coffee? Turn on the TV? To set the tone for a peaceful day, try to create a moment of peace right when you wake up. I like to begin my day with a cup of hot water with lemon. It gets your system going and is great for your digestive system. It's also great for your metabolism and helps to clear your skin! I'll take my lemon water to my yoga mat and begin from there.

When you're deep in your yoga practice you'll know what to do; it's all about being with the breath and working on what your body needs at that moment. If your hips are feeling tight, focus on that. Sore shoulders? Make that the center of your morning practice. You might feel a bit cold and stiff when you've just rolled out of bed, so a good idea is to always start your practice with a sequence to bring some heat into the body. When you are warm, your body will respond more readily. ✾

GREEN JUICE

*1 cucumber ✽ 2 cups spinach ✽ 2 cups kale
✽ 2 apples, cored ✽ 1 orange, peeled and
sectioned ✽ 1 lemon, peeled and sectioned
✽ 1 tablespoon chopped fresh gingerroot*

Add the ingredients to a masticating juicer one at a
time. Begin with the cucumber and use the apples
after the green leafy vegetables to make sure no
greens are left in the juicer.

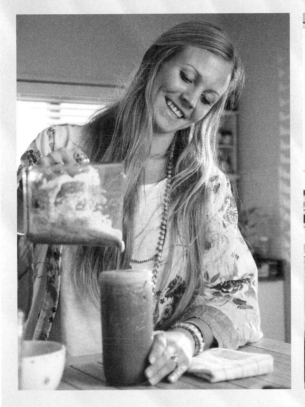

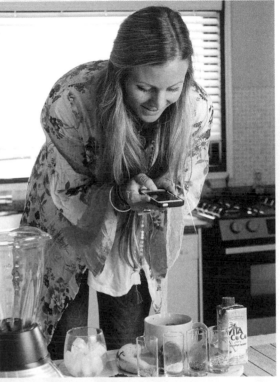

THE BIG GREEN SMOOTHIE

*1 banana ✽ 1 peach ✽ 2 cups kale ✽ 1 cup frozen
strawberries ✽ 1 cup coconut water ✽ Superfoods
of choice*

Add all of your ingredients into a high-speed blender
and blend. Add some ice at the very end to keep the
smoothie cold and delicious.

Suggested superfoods are hemp protein, chia
seeds, and maca powder (1 teaspoon of each).
Choose whichever you like!

---

*A centrifugal juicer works great for
juicing fruits, but if you can, invest
in a masticating juicer instead. The
masticating juicer doesn't make as much
noise and it's much more effective for
juicing greens like spinach and kale. Also,
centrifugal juicers heat your produce
slightly in the process, which lowers
the nutritional value of your juice.*

WHEN YOU FIRST START PRACTICING YOGA REGULARLY, YOU'LL HAVE SOME IMPORTANT REALIZATIONS:

1. This is much harder than I thought.

2. It also feels much better than I thought.

3. My body and my mind sometimes—or most of the time—completely disagree with each other, and the two sides of my body are very different.

4. How did I live my whole life without knowing how to breathe properly?

5. I want to do more of this.

AND IF YOU PRACTICE LONG ENOUGH YOU MIGHT EVEN REALIZE:

6. The clothes I wear have little to no effect on how well I perform on my yoga mat.

7. My body is connected to my emotions. My emotions are connected to my thoughts. My thoughts are connected to my ability to stay present. And my ability to stay present is connected to my body.

8. The poses we practice are not the destination, but the path.

9. The more I advance in my practice, the more I realize I have not advanced at all.

10. I want more of this.

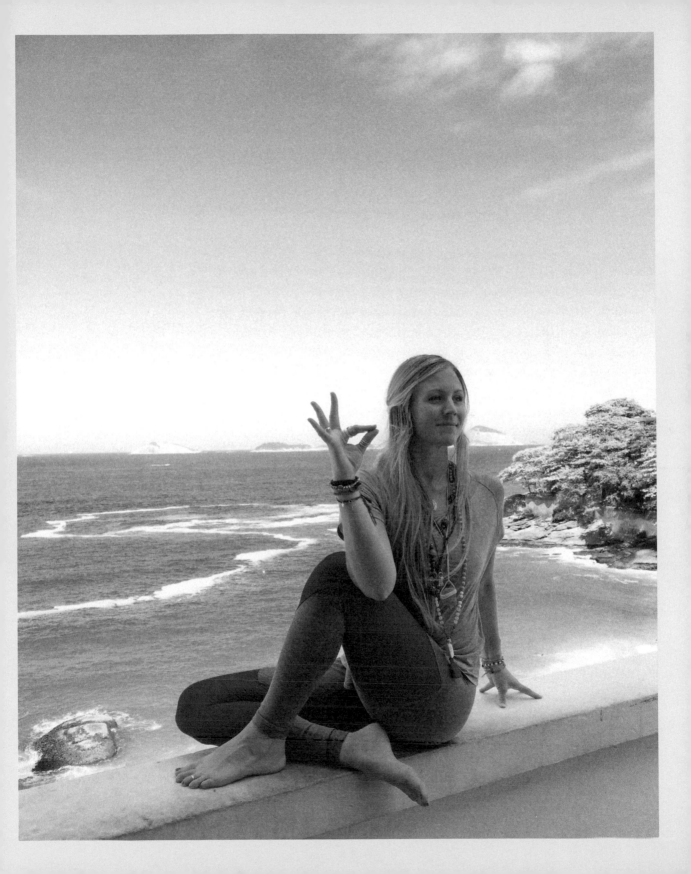

Sun Salutations—
The Perfect Morning Sequence

The Sun Salutation—in Sanskrit, Surya Namaskar—is a great way to create heat and serves as one of the foundational sequences of a yoga practice. You'll find it in many styles of yoga, mainly in flow classes such as Ashtanga and Vinyasa Flow. Take time to properly learn the poses (even if you're a seasoned practitioner) to ensure that you avoid injury and stay healthy in your practice. Always keep the integrity of the pose and learn proper alignment right away. Pay attention to what the pose feels like in your body so you'll know if you're overdoing something; back off or soften the pose when needed. Depending on how much you are looking to sweat and flow on your mat, do more or fewer Sun Salutations! If I'm short on time I'll roll out my mat and simply do ten Sun Salutations. This sequence has everything: chest expansion, forward folds, core work, upper body strengthening, heart opening, hamstring lengthening. When done properly, it's a very well-rounded aspect of your practice. And a great way to start the day!

"Begin where you are.
Use what you have. Do what you can."

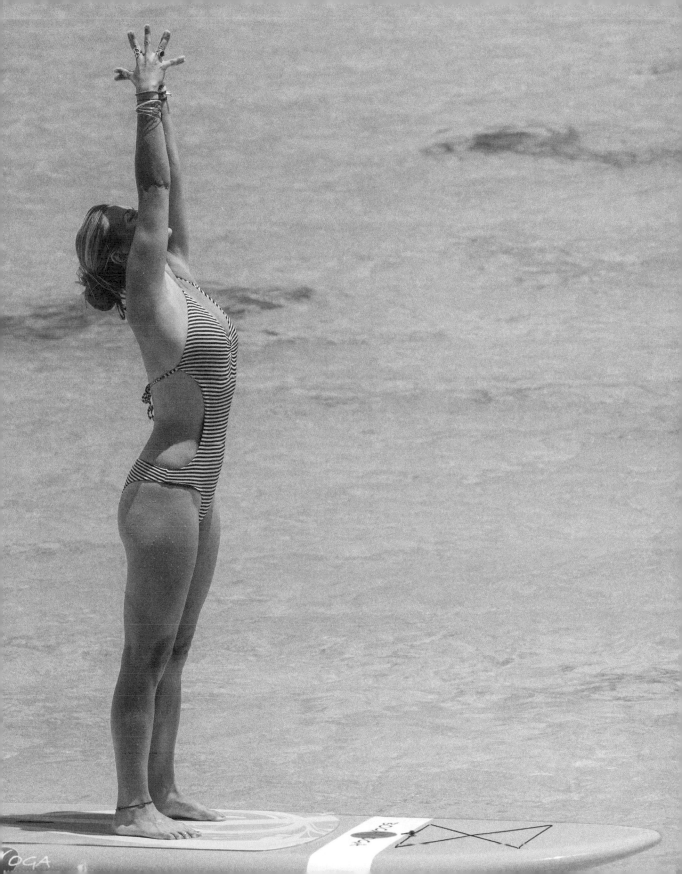

SURYA NAMASKAR A / SUN SALUTATION A

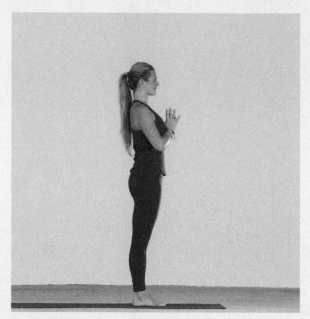

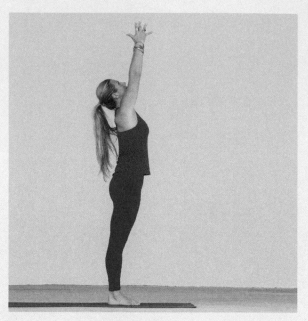

1 Come to a standing position with your two big toes connected, a slight space between your heels. Connect your hands to your heart center. Firmly ground your feet to the mat and feel the crown of your head drawing upward toward the sky. Exhale to bring your arms down by your side.

2 Soften the upper back and neck as you inhale and reach your arms up toward the sky. Engage your legs and lift up through the arches of the feet.

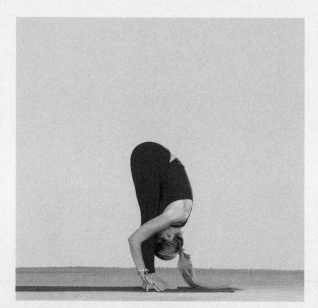

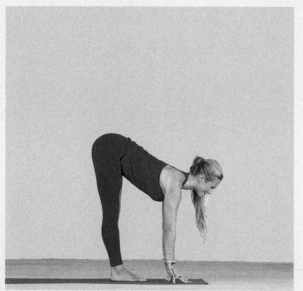

3 Exhale and fold forward, letting your body melt down toward the earth. If your hands don't reach the floor, bend your knees slightly. Relax the back of your neck and shift some weight into the balls of your feet.

4 Inhale to lengthen the spine, coming into a flat back, looking slightly forward. Activate your thighs to lift out of your kneecaps.

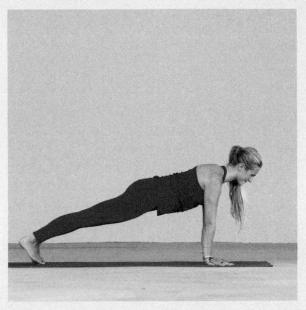

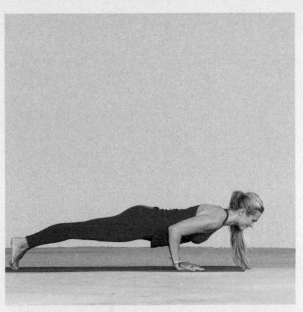

5 Exhale to step back one foot at a time, making your way to plank pose. With shoulders aligned right above your wrists, engage your core and press the floor away from you to avoid sinking into the shoulders.

6 Inhale and shift your weight slightly forward, then exhale to bend the elbows, lowering into Chaturanga Dandasana. Your shoulders should align with the elbows and the elbows should line up with the wrists. Think about absorbing the lower ribs and elongating the tailbone toward the heels.

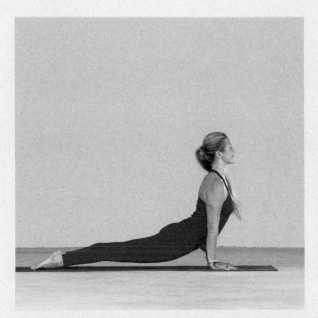

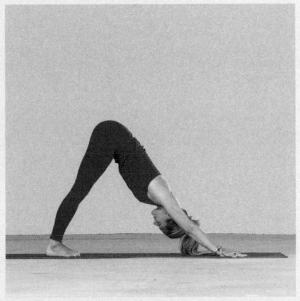

7 Inhale and press the balls of the feet toward the back of the mat, rolling over the toes into Upward-Facing Dog. Broaden through the collarbones, lift from the heart, and feel the shoulders sliding down the back.

8 Exhale to tuck your toes under, engaging your core to make your way back to Downward-Facing Dog. Rotate the inner thighs back, press the thumb and the index fingers down, and wrap the triceps back. Soften the neck and draw the heels toward the mat. Stay here for five deep, slow breaths.

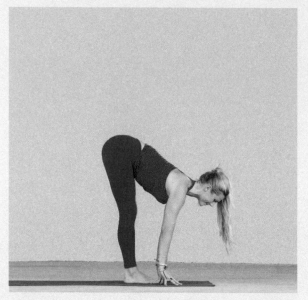

9 Look forward, bend your knees, and bring your hips back to prepare for your transition forward. On an exhale, step or lightly jump to the top of the mat. Inhale to lengthen the spine, gazing slightly forward.

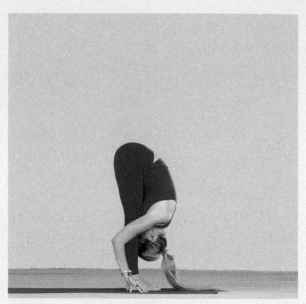

10 Exhale and fold forward.

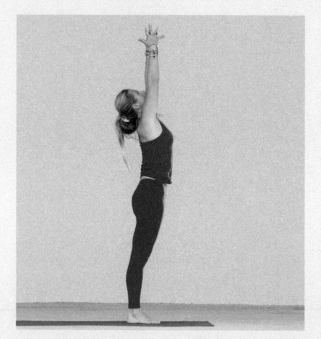

11 Inhale to root down through the feet, rising all the way up, stretching your fingers toward the sky.

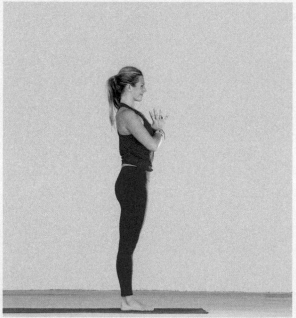

12 Exhale, bringing your hands to your heart center.

LOVING INSIGHTS

卐 In silence, breakthroughs come.

卐 Balance is the accumulated moments of presence and gratitude that you create throughout your day.

卐 Learn to act instead of reacting.

卐 Start where you are. Use what you have. Do what you can.

STARTING YOUR DAY OFF RIGHT

卐 Don't keep your phone in the bedroom—get an old-school alarm clock if you need one. The first thing you do in the morning should not include social media or e-mails!

卐 Drink hot water with lemon when you first wake up to cleanse your system.

卐 Practice yoga before breakfast. Everything you do counts! Decide to do fifteen minutes of gentle stretching, some dynamic Sun Salutations, or just a simple meditation. The important thing is to give yourself time on the mat every day. If you have an hour to spare, treat yourself to a full hour on the mat!

卐 Decide what time your active workday begins. Keep away from pointless scrolling during the first hours of the day. Read a book. Make a beautiful breakfast. Spend time with your family. If you allow your mornings to be sacred, it will set the tone for the rest of your day.

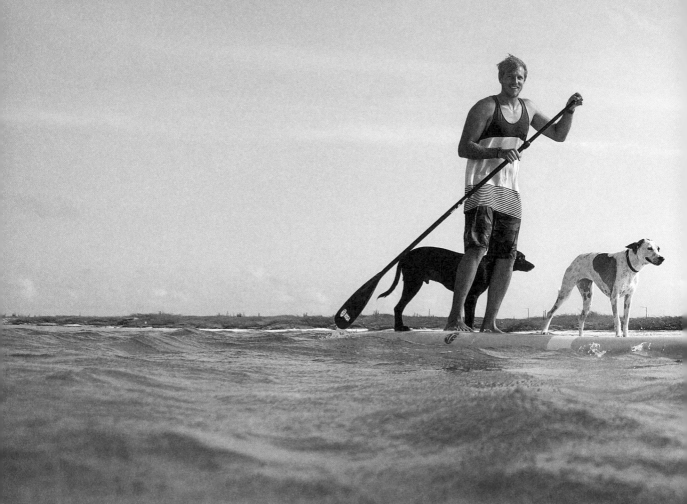

CHAPTER 2

To love what is ahead, you must love what has come before

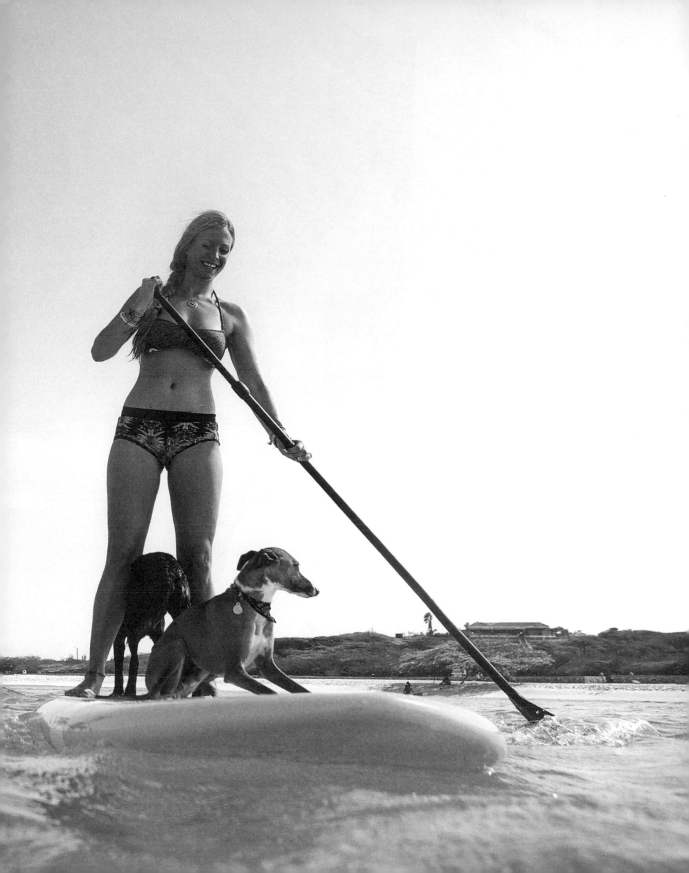

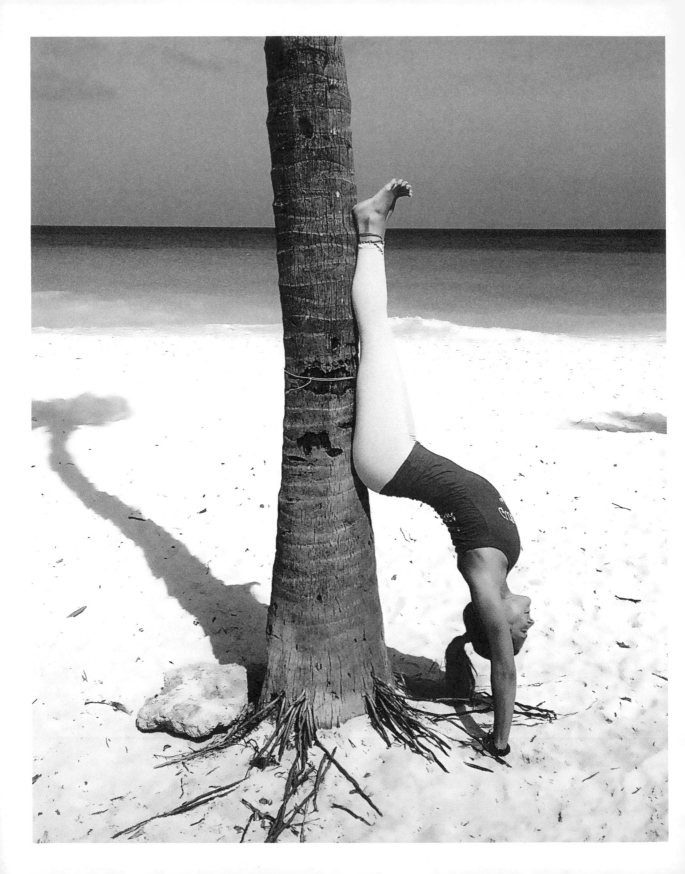

It's been a long journey to get to where I am today. I wasn't a naturally balanced person growing up, and I was lucky to find yoga at the young age of seventeen. I took my first yoga class in Thailand, while I was on vacation with my family. The class was led by a small Thai man, and I remember being struck by how calm and peaceful he was. We were on bamboo mats in the shade and he led us through different poses while instructing us to inhale and exhale. I'd never experienced anything like it, and even though the class didn't change my life or my view of the world, I left feeling invigorated and happy. I was not a happy teenager, and I was still about two years away from taking my first steps toward making yoga a substantial part of my life.

When I was little, my family moved a lot. My parents split up when I was only two years old, and as often happens with couples who separate, there was a lot of drama. During this period my brother and I moved back and forth between my parents. Eventually my mom met and fell in love with a man who was a fighter pilot for the Swedish army, and for a year or two we led very quiet lives. My brother and I went to day care, we lived in just one place, and my grandmother was with us a lot. We would all go skiing every chance we got and spent lots of time in the mountains. One of my clearest memories is watching my stepdad hack out a little cave in the snow, using his ski to dig us a cozy place out of the side of the slope where we sat and drank hot chocolate. Also, sitting on his shoulders singing along to the live band at the lodge after skiing. The song was "What's Up?" by 4 Non Blondes; and every time I hear that song I think of him and our lives at that time. These were some of the happiest days of my childhood.

Of course, good things sometimes come to an end. Just a day after my mom and stepdad signed the contract for our new house, his plane crashed into the ocean and our lives changed drastically. I was only five years old.

His death was a defining moment in my life. My mother lost the love of her life, my little brother and I lost our stepdad, and again our lives were turned upside down, but on a level we had never experienced before. The years that followed were extremely dark and difficult, and even though my mom did her best to take care of us, I had to grow up fast. I hardly have any memories at all from when I was five until I was about ten years old. I'd remember fragments here and there, but some were so vague I didn't know if they were from a dream I once had or if they were real. I remember my grand-

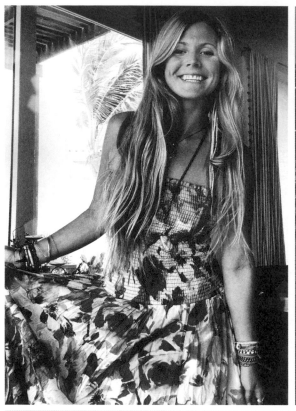
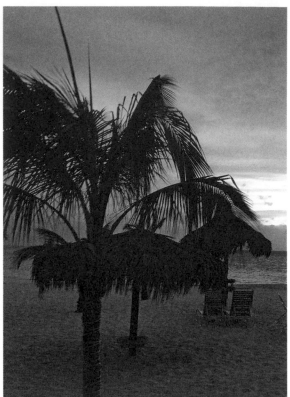
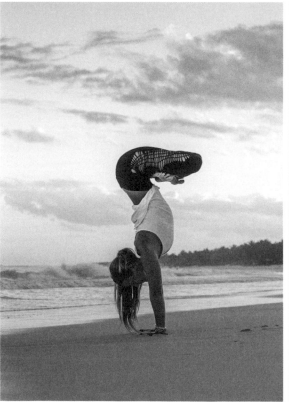
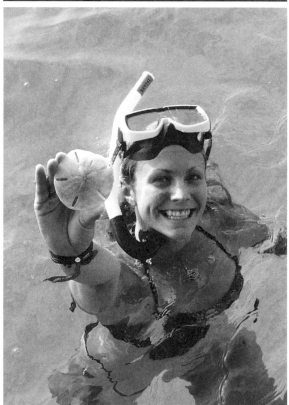

mother rushing my brother and me out of the church during the funeral, covering our ears so we couldn't hear my mother's screams. I remember sad, sad faces everywhere we went. Lots of candy and presents from relatives and people I didn't know. People, everywhere, all the time. We had to leave our apartment in the south of Sweden. Time passed, and then all of a sudden we were alone. The three of us: me, my little brother, my mom. The situation was too painful for us to discuss; we stopped talking about my stepdad, and my mother was too fragile to answer my questions.

"Where did he go?" I'd ask over and over again. My mother always turned her face away. One day someone else answered me: "He went to heaven." "Why?" I said. I didn't know where heaven was and why he would choose to go there without us. "Well, he loved you and your brother so, so much, and when he was flying he was rushing home to see you. But he flew too fast and crashed his plane, so now he is in heaven and you have to be strong for your mother."

I don't know who told me this, if it was a relative or a friend of the family, but this scarred me so deeply it would take me more than a decade to even understand. I was just five years old, lost and alone, looking for someone to comfort me. And I find out my stepdad left us to go to heaven—because I made him hurry? I couldn't wrap my five-year-old brain around this, and I decided it was all my fault. If it hadn't been for me, he would still be here, and my mom wouldn't be sad all the time. This is when my memory starts to get very, very fuzzy. I remember walking into my mother's bedroom to wake her up every morning, always finding her facedown with a pillow covering the back of her head. I asked her why she did that, and she told me it helped her fall asleep. For the longest time I slept with a pillow covering my face, thinking it would help me fall asleep easier, too. Now I know she wasn't sleeping, but bawling into the mattress at night so we wouldn't hear her scream. I remember holding my brother's hand while we walked to school, making sure he didn't trip on the sidewalk. I remember my sixth birthday party. An ambulance. More screaming. Suddenly living with my dad in a house we didn't really know. I remember going to see my mom in the hospital, lots of crying and her hugging me so hard I couldn't breathe. I didn't find the suicide letters she left us until much later.

It wasn't until I got on the spiritual path in my late teens and started inquiring about this time that some memories came back to me. I've learned that sometimes the

"Our spiritual journey begins the day we decide to come to terms with our past."

---

mind does what it has to do to keep us alive. Massive trauma is simply too much for our hearts to handle, so the mind shuts down to protect us. Time passes and we forget. But the difficulties we experience shape us, and our spiritual journey begins the day we decide to come to terms with our past. For me, my parents' divorce, my stepdad's death, and my mother's suicide attempt were the most significant things that ever happened in my life. I didn't know it then, of course, but a time would come when I would be able to look back and feel grateful for my childhood.

For my family, the pain subsided after a few years and we eventually moved on, but it took a very long time for my mom to recover and become whole again. She was twenty-five years old when the accident happened, around my age right now, and I cannot even for a second imagine what life would be like if I lost my husband. I don't know if I'd survive, and I pray I will never, ever have to find out. My mother overcame a loss greater than I could possibly ever understand, and with time, she healed and found love again. She was the one who nudged me in the right direction, the one who never stopped fighting for us all, and even though we all went through some extremely difficult times, I know she did the absolute best she could with what she had. I admire my mother for making it through that time and for blossoming into the strong, confident, happy woman she is today. I now have four sisters in addition to my brother, and I know the things we went through growing up helped shape us into the people we are. When all of this happened I was still a child, and my journey had just begun.

We had lived in more than ten different places by the time I was twelve. I lived mostly with my mother but spent weekends and vacations with my dad, who lived in Latvia and Spain. My parents both had new lives; they both remarried and had two more kids each—in the same year. When my dad married Inga, who would become my stepmother, I spoke in front of two hundred people. The first line of my speech was "The year 2000 was the year my parents finally got married. Except not to each other." The crowd laughed, and so did I. My mom and dad were on good terms, I had stability in my life, and we had made it through the dark. Everything was okay.

When I became a teenager, my life changed again. This time it wasn't my parents splitting up, but my mom and her new husband, as well as my dad and his new wife. I was older this time around and had small sisters to care for, and when divorce struck our family again, it angered me. *What is wrong with my parents?* I thought. There were

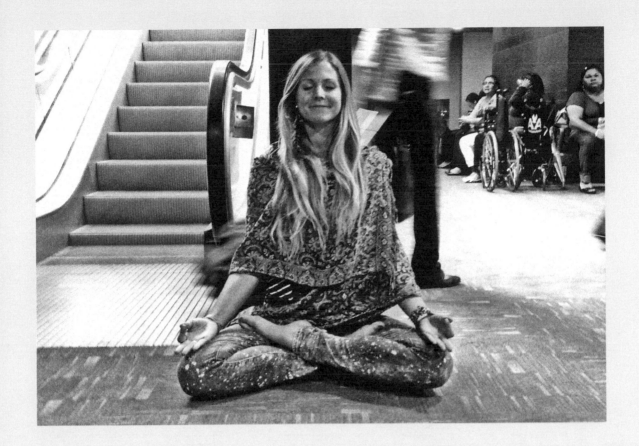

BREATHING

When practicing yoga and meditation you want to focus your awareness inward and deeply connect to the breath. The breath is the core of your yoga practice and a beautiful way to stay connected to the body. If you find yourself losing the connection to the breath or having a difficult time breathing, it might mean you've gone too deeply into a pose and your body is telling you to back off slightly or just slow down a little bit.

Keep the breath flowing in and out of the nose and try to find a balance between the two sides of the breath, with the inhales and exhales equal in length. Direct your inhales down toward the bottom of the lungs, feeling the lower belly expand. Notice how the low belly contracts again as you exhale, emptying the lungs. Keep a steady pace of breath, letting the sound of your breathing help you maintain focus as you practice.

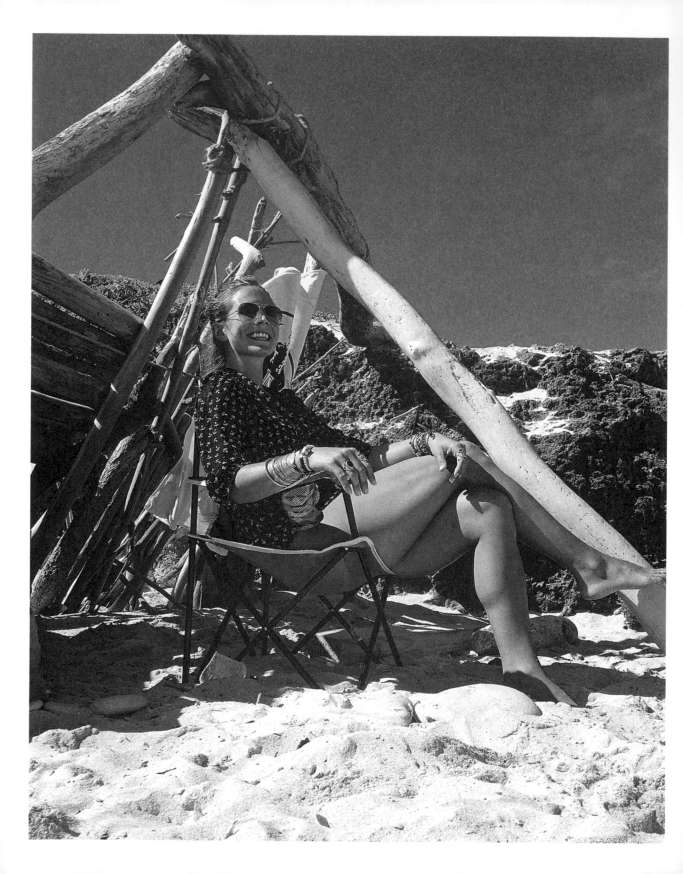

"Since I couldn't manage the chaos I felt within and the chaos at home, I started creating more of it wherever I went."

---

little kids to care for! I took it upon myself to be responsible for their well-being. Of course I failed. I couldn't be a mom and a dad and a big sister all at once—and no one had even asked me to! I felt it was my job to ensure that everyone was happy and to make sure my mom was okay. When the pressure of it all became too much, I started turning away from my family and toward other things. Since I couldn't manage the chaos I felt within and the chaos at home, I started creating more of it wherever I went.

I think I was thirteen when all of a sudden I became really "cool." So cool I refused to get braces even though I needed them badly (so badly that I ended up getting them when I was sixteen instead, which was much worse!). I started shoplifting and drinking on the weekends and also picked up the terrible habit of smoking. I thought smoking was awesome. It gave me a crowd, a reputation, and a feeling of *screw you all—I can do whatever I want*. I wanted control of my own life and smoking was a way for me to do that. I got addicted fast, physically and socially, and I smoked about a pack a day until I turned seventeen. Of course, smoking and the severe asthma I'd suffered from since I was little didn't really go hand in hand—not even a little. In the beginning I was okay, but it soon became normal for me to sneak outside, take a puff from my inhaler, and then light a cigarette. To this day, I can hardly believe it. I became an expert liar, telling my parents elaborate stories about sitting in cafés with my friends (you were allowed to smoke indoors at the time, so I said that's why I always reeked of smoke), about friends who smoked (I would NEVER!), I had lit incense and it just has a similar scent, someone lit candles, there was a fire—you name it. I never, ever admitted I was a smoker. Of course they figured it out eventually, but there was nothing they could do. I was a mess. My mom would ground me for months at a time; I'd jump out the window. They'd take my allowance away; I'd shoplift. They threatened to send me to boarding school; I ran away from home, slept at the train station in downtown Stockholm for two nights, and didn't return until they begged me to come back. I remember my dad lecturing me with tears in his eyes ("Don't you understand you can die?"), but it didn't even faze me. I thought smoking was a part of my identity, and I wasn't prepared to let that go.

It started with cigarettes but went on to alcohol (a lot) and also drugs. I had older boyfriends and I started hanging out with bad people doing bad things. It wasn't good,

૭ Make peace with your past. Come to terms with the difficulties you've been through. It's the only way to create a peaceful life.

૭ Forgiveness is the key to happiness.

૭ The most important thing is not what happens to you in life but how you choose to react to what's happening. Life is not as serious as your mind makes it out to be. Learn to create distance between your perception of the world and what's actually going on in the present moment, instead of simply reacting blindly to those things that come your way. Stay present and live in the moment.

૭ It doesn't matter where you come from or what you've experienced in your past. Your happiness is in your hands! We are not victims of our circumstances. We have the power to change how we are feeling.

૭ Life happens for you—not to you.

૭ Think about what you are carrying with you from your past. What patterns and behaviors have you picked up that maybe don't match the person you actually are deep down?

૭ Tell yourself: *I will not create any more drama in my life.* Make yourself the promise to live a good life!

૭ Whom do you need to forgive? Remember that you are the only one suffering by clinging to the past. Forgive everyone for everything for your own sake.

૭ Do more of the things that make you smile. Focus on being happy!

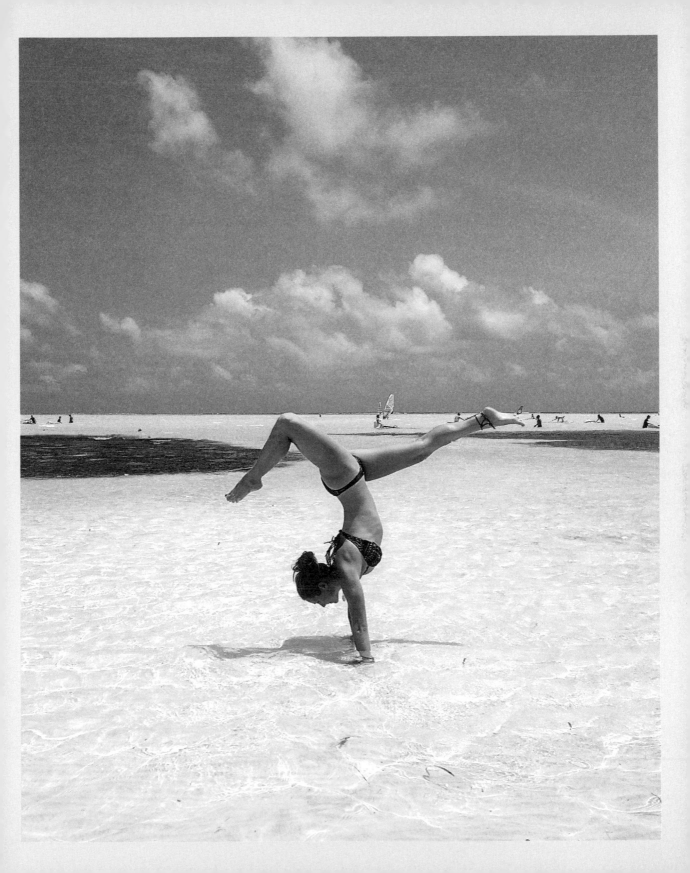

and worst of all was the lying. I lied about everything. I lied so much I couldn't even remember what was true anymore. I lied about where I was, who I was with, what I was doing. I remember my mom telling me: "I would rather have you do drugs and tell me where you are than have you drink a beer and lie about where you are. At least then I would know where to go to save you when things go really wrong." And she meant it. She had absolutely no idea where I was most of the time or how she could help me.

I was only thirteen the first time I had to be driven to the emergency room with alcohol poisoning. I had taken the red line subway back and forth (the end of the red line in Stockholm was not the best neighborhood for a passed-out thirteen-year-old girl at the time), had thrown up all over myself, had been robbed, and finally was found by a friend who called my mom. I remember hanging my head over the toilet, thinking I was going to die. I was also thirteen when I got my first tattoo, simply as a response to my dad saying "over my dead body" after I'd jokingly told him I wanted to get one. I didn't even want a tattoo, I just wanted to do the exact opposite of what everybody expected of me. I started spending time in bad parts of Stockholm. Thinking of it now—I was so young! I was just a child. But I was determined to be destructive, and there was nothing my parents could do to stop me.

At fourteen I got high on something bad, thinking it was weed, and ended up walking from Hornstull to northern Lidingö (if you're from Stockholm, you know how far this is). It wasn't until I woke up the next day with my sheets stained with blood that I realized I'd been walking barefoot. In October. This was also the age I was when I told my mom I hated her for the first time. I started stealing alcohol from my parents. I quickly figured out how to replace vodka with water in the bottles no one ever touched, and when I got caught doing that and my parents completely stopped keeping alcohol in the house, I got a fake ID.

At fifteen I went to Spain with a few girlfriends. We partied for a week straight, and one night someone slipped something in my drink at a bar in Puerto Banús. The doorman put me into a taxi and called the security at our house to make sure someone would let me in, as I'd lost my purse and my keys. This was the first of three times in my young teens that I got drugged (probably with the intention of rape). I was always incredibly lucky that nothing worse happened to me than excessive vomiting and hangovers that lasted for weeks. I finally learned to never accept drinks from anyone (not

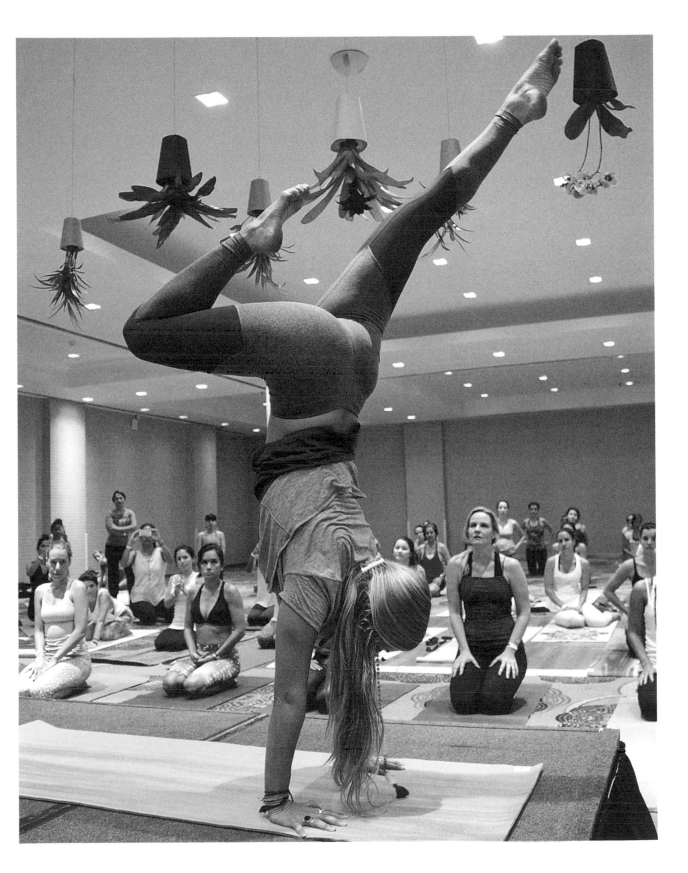

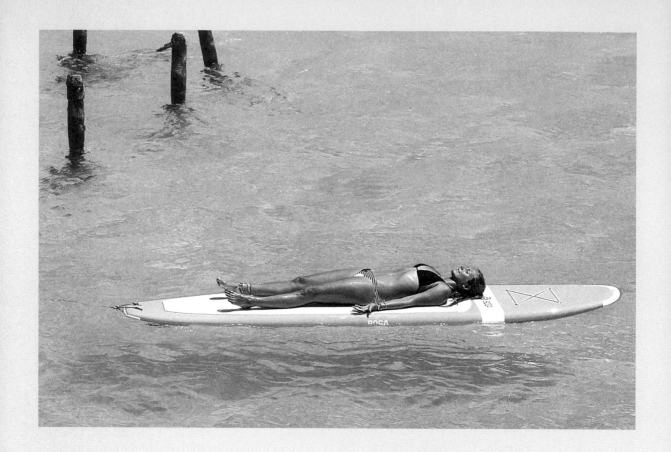

CORPSE POSE / SAVASANA

꩜ Finish every yoga class with Savasana, Corpse Pose, and allow the body to relax. It's in Savasana, a beautiful place of silence and presence, that we get to soak up all the yumminess of our hard work on the mat.

꩜ Lie on your back with your arms down by your sides, palms facing up. If your lower back is sensitive, you can place a bolster or a pillow beneath your knees for support. I like to burn some palo santo, holy wood, right before Savasana to raise the vibration in the room and inspire total relaxation (plus it smells amazing!). Close your eyes, let your body soften, and feel the weight of your body melting into the floor. Release any control you might have had over your breath throughout the practice and come back to the natural pace of your inhales and exhales. Follow the breath every step of the way, and embrace the softness of the breath that arises when you let everything be. Stay present. For every hour of yoga you've practiced, stay in Savasana for ten minutes or more. When you're ready, roll over to your right side. Your heart is on your left, so when you "come back to life" from Corpse Pose, you rise with the heart first, always letting your heart lead the way. In yoga class you will often hear your teacher say "Namaste" at the end of practice—say "Namaste" back! The word means "The light within me honors the light within you," a sacred way to show reverence and respect.

even from bartenders) and to always order bottled drinks, covering the spout with my thumb.

At sixteen, I got pulled over for drunk driving and had to spend the night in jail. I got out, picked up some beer, and went right back to the party. This is also how old I was when my boyfriend hit me for the first time. I started spending a lot of time at a bar in downtown Stockholm, and after we got to know the staff, they stopped asking us for IDs, assuming we were eighteen (the legal drinking age in Sweden). One evening my oldest friend in the world was walking home from a party and found me passed out in the snow next to the road. He brought me home, cooked me food, drew me a bath, and made me promise to stop drinking, or we couldn't stay friends anymore. We had a fight and didn't speak to each other for a year. I didn't stop drinking. By this point I had already been drinking and going to clubs for years and was known as the go-to girl at school if you wanted to party. I was angry and insecure, doing all I could to draw attention to myself.

At seventeen, I was out partying and got in a car with a drunk driver. Driving ninety miles per hour he rammed into another car and we skidded off the highway, flipped over several times, and finally smashed into a tree, landing upside down. I got away with a few broken ribs and internal bleeding. I drank every single day. Every day. I finally stopped lying to my mom, but only because I think we both stopped caring. At eighteen I gave up. At high school graduation in Sweden, it's traditional to dress up in white and celebrate in the park outside the school together with friends and teachers. Everybody was there in the grass, signing one another's graduation hats, hugging and singing. I sat in my friend Jack's old Volvo parked in the back of the parking lot, drinking vodka straight from the bottle and wishing for it all to be over.

At one point in the middle of all this, my grandmother died. My grandmother had been the only constant in my life, the sensible, calm, caring person who always knew the right thing to say. When she passed away I hit a new low and my family finally had had enough. I'd spent years lying, fighting, stealing money, and creating more chaos than they had ever seen before. Even I started to get the uneasy feeling that maybe things wouldn't ever be okay again.

My mom could have thrown me out of the house. She could have let me clean up my own mess. She could have given up on me completely. But she didn't. *She sent me off to a therapeutic meditation retreat.* I don't know how on earth she convinced me to go, but one day I found myself on a train going up to a small town in northern Sweden to spend a week at a meditation center. I was terrified. No, scratch that. I was beyond terrified. Out of all the things I had done—and at eighteen I had already done it all—this was more out of my comfort zone than anything I could possibly imagine. Meditate? Me? I had taken that one yoga class in Thailand while we were there on vacation, but that was it. I had never meditated. All I knew was cigarettes and beer and fighting with people. Jealous, hot-tempered, and impatient, I had turned into an incredibly difficult person. I thought life was about living as fast as possible, and looking good while doing it. A lot of my time was spent fixing my makeup, buying new clothes, and coming up with new ways to sneak into the hottest clubs downtown. Meditating had never even crossed my mind. So when I got off the train and into the cab that was going to take me to the meditation center, I broke down, started crying, and told the cabdriver to turn around. The cabbie looked me in the eye and said, "I think you should give it a try. I've seen many people throughout the years get off the train looking just as nervous as you, but they all come back smiling, looking very calm. Here, take my number. If it's really bad and you want to leave after one day, call me and I'll drive you to the train."

I took his number, and he dropped me off at the center. This was the start of a whole new life for me.

For the first time, I learned how to quiet my mind. Twice a day we had group meditations and therapeutic sessions, and in between there was absolute silence. No phones, no computers, no talking. Just silence. I had never been silent in my entire life before. In the sessions I was given tools to deal with my past, and I started working through the issues causing my anger and resentment. I realized I hadn't mourned the death of my stepfather—even though I was only five years old, I'd been so busy taking care of my mom and my little brother that I never allowed myself to be sad. No one talked about it in the family and it was like a chapter of my life was torn out of the big book of our family. I had a lot of grief inside of me that I'd never gotten the chance to release. And anger. Oh, boy, was I angry. I was angry at my mother for being so fragile when I was little. I was angry at my father for being distant. I was angry at myself!

My entire view of the world changed in just one week, and I left the center a different version of myself. I realized that I had taken on traits that were not at all who

I really was at my core. I wasn't an angry person. Situations and events that came my way had made me into an angry person. When I learned how to let go of those events, I could let go of my anger and stop feeling mad all the time! I got a glimpse into what life could be like if I wasn't so preoccupied with smoking and drinking myself to death. I started looking at the big picture, and all of a sudden, I realized that I wanted to be happy. I'd never had a longing like that before in my life. I'd been too busy just surviving, but now that I had tools to deal with all the feelings I had locked up inside, I wanted more. I wanted happiness. Balance. Peace.

Looking back at it now, I didn't have a terrible time growing up at all; I had two parents that did their absolute best with what they had. Most of the negative situations I found myself in, I created on my own. I came home and had a big talk with my parents. I quit smoking. I stopped drinking. I started going outside, being in nature, and I started spending time with different people. I went back to the meditation center one more time, this time for ten full days, for a deeper course on how to resolve childhood issues. This one was, if possible, even more profound for me, and I found myself changing more and more. It wasn't so much that I was becoming a different person—quite the opposite. I was chipping away at the marble to find the masterpiece hidden beneath all the experiences I had accumulated throughout my life. I was becoming myself.

It might sound crazy, but it really was as if a veil had been lifted. There was a wisdom deep inside me that I'd never known before, and life didn't feel all that difficult anymore. I started meditating daily and began devouring spiritual books. Because I had changed so much, many of my friends changed along with me. Instead of being "that crazy party girl," I became "that crazy hippie girl," and my friends started to come to me for advice. I was feeling much, much happier than I ever had before, but I didn't have a community. No one I knew was interested in meditation or spirituality. I realized that in order to delve deeper into this new way of living, I had to go on a journey to find like-minded people. I knew I had barely scratched the surface, and I wanted more.

So I booked a ticket to Costa Rica. ✸

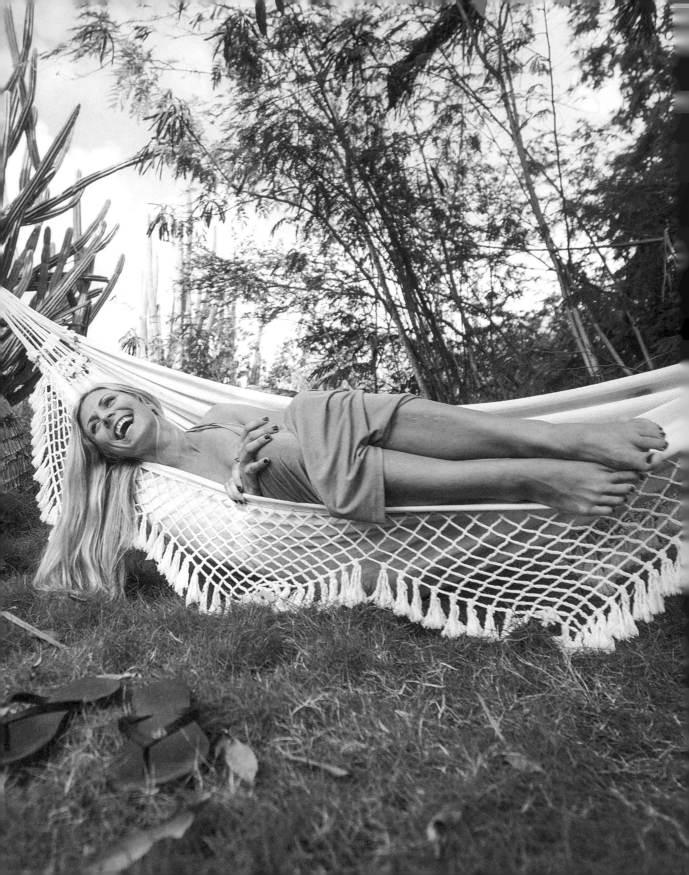

RAW AVOCADO SOUP

2 avocados ❦ ½ broccoli crown ❦ 1 cup spinach ❦ 1 small chunk yellow onion ❦ 1 clove garlic, minced ❦ Salt and pepper to taste ❦ ½ red bell pepper, chopped (for garnish)

Place all of the ingredients except the bell pepper in a blender. Go easy with the onion and the garlic—start with half of each and then slowly add slightly more to taste. When blended, the onion can become slightly overpowering, so a little bit will go a long way. Add just enough hot water to get the blender going and start blending. Add more hot water little by little until you have the perfect consistency for your soup. Taste and add more onion and garlic if needed. Add more salt and pepper, if necessary, and serve with pieces of chopped bell pepper for garnish.

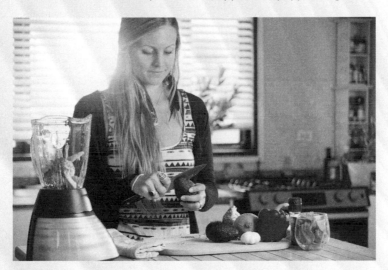

SUPERFOOD SALAD

2 tablespoons olive oil ❦ 1 cup chopped shiitake mushrooms ❦ 1 bunch asparagus spears, halved ❦ 1 pound fresh sugar snap peas ❦ 1 clove garlic, minced ❦ Salt and pepper to taste ❦ 1 cup baby spinach ❦ 1 cup shredded red cabbage ❦ 1 cup shredded kale ❦ 1 cup shelled and cooked edamame ❦ ½ cup chopped radishes ❦ 1 avocado, peeled and cubed ❦ ½ cup alfalfa sprouts ❦ 1 cup blueberries ❦ ½ cup pumpkin seeds ❦ Pomegranate seeds (for garnish) ❦ Chia seeds (for garnish)

In a large skillet, heat the olive oil. Pan-fry the shiitake mushrooms, the asparagus, and the sugar snap peas together with the garlic and salt and pepper. Put aside and let cool. Mix the remaining vegetables in a big bowl. Add the blueberries and pumpkin seeds. Mix everything together with the pan-fried vegetables, add the dressing, and garnish with pomegranate seeds and chia seeds. Enjoy!

CARROT DRESSING

2 big carrots, chopped. ❦ 1 inch fresh gingerroot, peeled and chopped ❦ 2 cloves garlic, minced ❦ 2 teaspoons apple cider vinegar ❦ 2 tablespoons honey ❦ Juice of 1 lemon ❦ ¼ cup olive oil

Boil the carrots in a small saucepan until soft. Drain but keep the water. Mix the carrots with the ginger, garlic, vinegar, honey, lemon juice, and olive oil. Add water from the carrots until the dressing is the proper consistency.

Dressing will last 3 to 4 days in the refrigerator.

LOVE WHAT HAS COME BEFORE

Twists, Hips,
and Hamstrings

Certain areas of our bodies tend to become very stiff after a long night's sleep or a day at the office, or simply from the repetitive movement of day-to-day living. I love working with twists, hip openers, and poses that stretch the back of the legs. I usually move through these stretches in the morning after my Sun Salutations or in the evening before I go to bed. When you've opened up and softened the body with these exercises, you'll feel so much more relaxed!

Twists are very cleansing; you are wringing out the spine in the same way you wring out a wet towel. Always move into twists gently, distributing the twisting action evenly throughout the spine, listening to the body. Start softly and deepen when it's appropriate. A good rule of thumb is to only twist to the point where you can maintain a deep and full breath. If your breathing feels restricted, back off slightly and return to the breath.

When it comes to the hip openers, let your body guide you and go only as deep as you feel comfortable. You never want pain or sharp sensation, and you want to make sure your knees are comfortable throughout. We usually hold a lot of tension and tightness in the hips, so if this is a part of the body that you know you need to work on, spend some extra time with these poses!

The hamstrings need the right kind of stretch—you want to feel the sensation in the belly of the muscle, never in the muscle attachments. Keep your feet active and use a yoga strap if you need to.

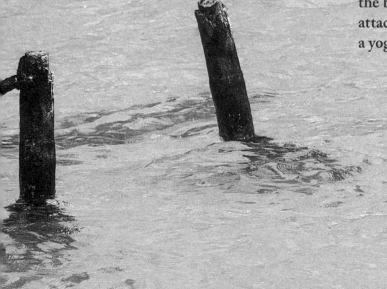

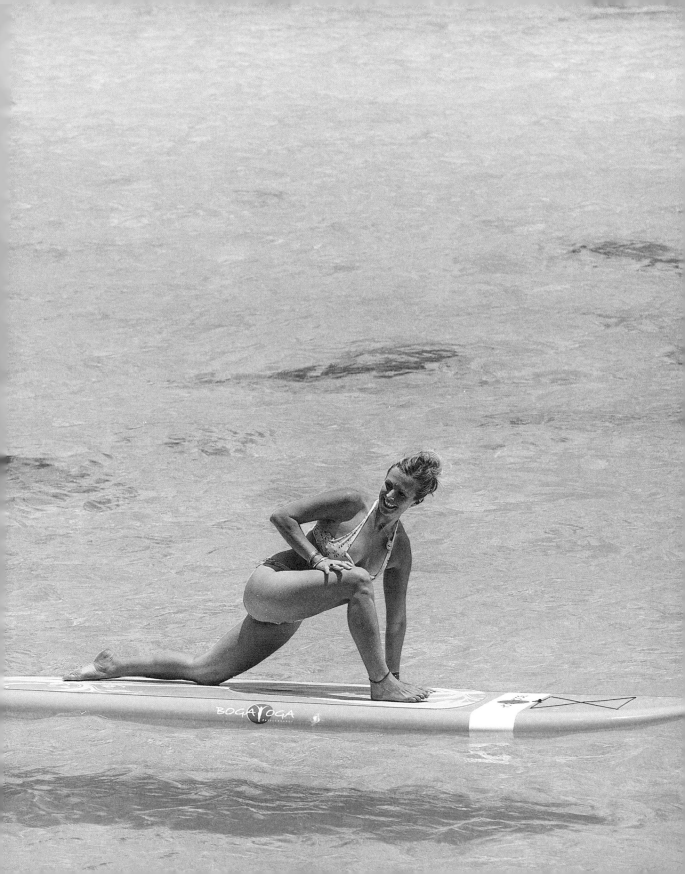

1. SUPTA PADANGUSTHASANA / RECLINING BIG TOE POSE

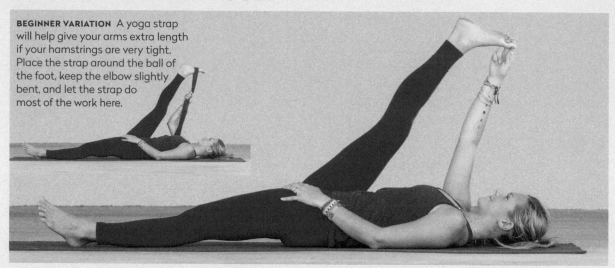

BEGINNER VARIATION A yoga strap will help give your arms extra length if your hamstrings are very tight. Place the strap around the ball of the foot, keep the elbow slightly bent, and let the strap do most of the work here.

Begin with the right leg. Lying on your back, extend the right leg straight up toward the sky. Hold on to the back of the thigh, the calf, the ankle, or the big toe, depending on what you're comfortable with. Your head should stay relaxed on the mat. Soften the shoulders, flex the right foot, and keep the toes active. Keep grounding the left leg to the earth. You want to feel a stretch at the back of the right leg, but never pain! Keep it at a level that is perfect for where you are. Stay for 10 to 15 slow, deep breaths.

2. SUPTA PADANGUSTHASANA, VARIATION

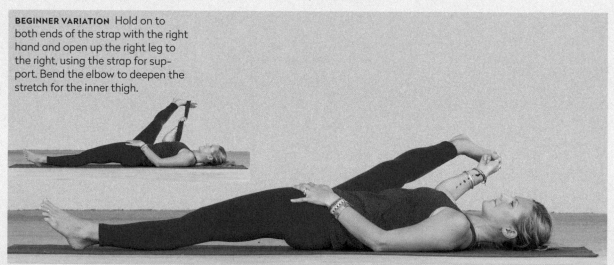

BEGINNER VARIATION Hold on to both ends of the strap with the right hand and open up the right leg to the right, using the strap for support. Bend the elbow to deepen the stretch for the inner thigh.

Place your left hand on the left hip for awareness and stability. Inhale to prepare and exhale to open up your right leg toward the right side. Engage the right thigh, and keep grounding the left hip to the earth. Keep the hips level and neutral; if your left hipbone starts to lift off the mat, you've gone too far! Stay for 10 to 15 slow, deep breaths.

3. SUPTA MATSYENDRASANA / SUPINE SPINAL TWIST

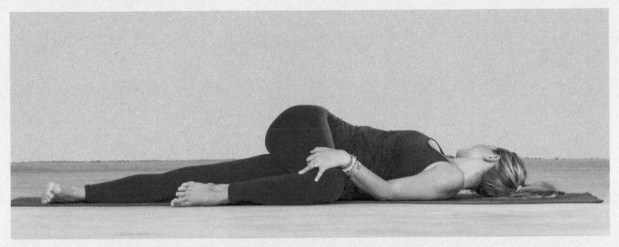

Engage the right leg to lift it up toward the sky. Bend the right knee in toward the chest and draw it over toward the left side of the body, coming into a twist. Roll over to the outer left hip and make sure the right shoulder stays grounded to the mat. Extend the right arm perpendicular to the body, keeping the palm of the hand facing upward. Gaze toward the right thumb if your neck allows. Stay for 10 breaths.

4. SUCIRANDHRASANA / THE EYE OF THE NEEDLE

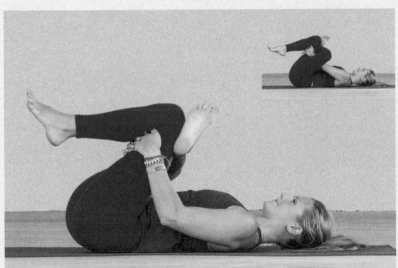

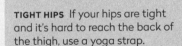

ADVANCED VARIATION If your hips are fairly open you can interlace your fingers on top of the left shinbone instead of at the back of the thigh. Gently guide the right elbow into the right knee to deepen the stretch, but make sure your knees are comfortable at all times.

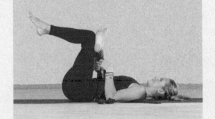

TIGHT HIPS If your hips are tight and it's hard to reach the back of the thigh, use a yoga strap.

Engage your core to untwist, bringing your gaze up first and then bringing the knee back into the chest. Place the sole of the left foot on the ground and place the right ankle above the left knee on the thigh. Flex the right foot and press the big toe away from the body. Interlace the fingers at the back of the left thigh, drawing the left leg in toward the chest to deepen the opening in the right hip. Lengthen the tailbone toward the mat and stay for 10 breaths. Do the full sequence (poses 1–4) on the opposite side of the body.

ARDHA MATSYENDRASANA / SEATED TWIST

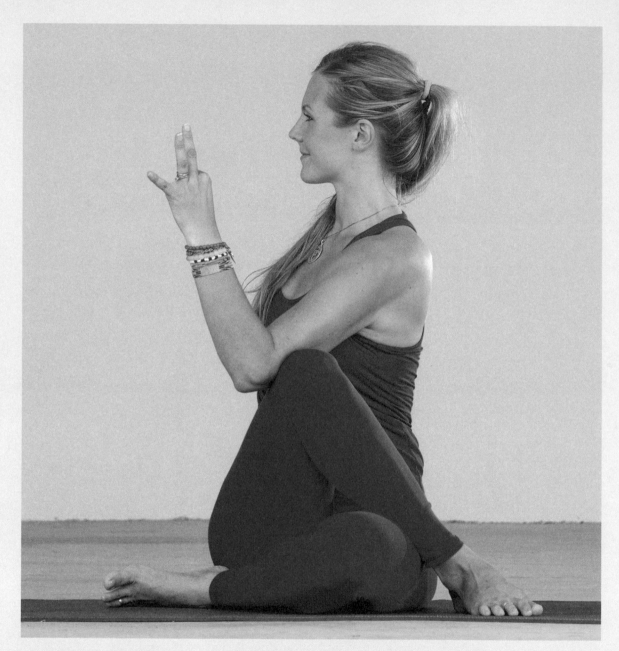

Come into a seated position with both legs extended straight in front of you. Bend the right knee, placing the sole of the foot on the mat by the inner left thigh. Cross the right leg over the left, now pressing the sole of the right foot into the mat outside the left leg. Bend the left knee so that the left heel ends up close to the outer hip. Start twisting toward the right, bringing the right hand behind you, fingertips pressing into the mat. Ground down through both sit bones and lengthen the crown of the head toward the sky. Place the left elbow to the outside of the right knee, gently deepening the twist. Gaze over the right shoulder. Stay for 5 deep breaths, untwist slowly, and repeat on the other side.

AGNISTAMBHASANA / DOUBLE PIGEON POSE

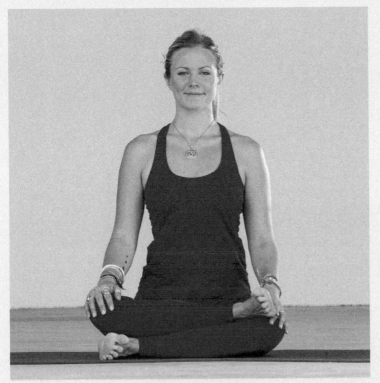

1 Come to a comfortable seated position. Place the left shinbone so that it's parallel to the edge of your mat, and then place the right ankle on top of the left knee and the right knee on top of the left ankle. You want the shins to stack on top of each other. Depending on your hips this may or may not be comfortable. If the top knee ends up very high above the ankle, fold up a blanket and place under the knee for support or come into the softer variation of Sukhasana (see below). The more the shinbones line up with the top of the mat, the deeper the stretch for the hips. Flex both your feet and press the inner border of the feet away from the body.

TIGHT HIPS Come to Sukhasana (Easy Pose), a comfortable seat with the right leg in front of the left.

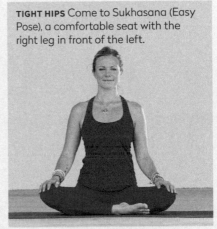

2 Inhale to lengthen the spine; exhale to fold forward while walking the fingertips forward and away from the body. Relax your neck, and if you have the space, find a place to rest your forehead—on a block or two, on top of your hands, or on the mat. Stay for 10 breaths and then repeat with the left leg on top of the right.

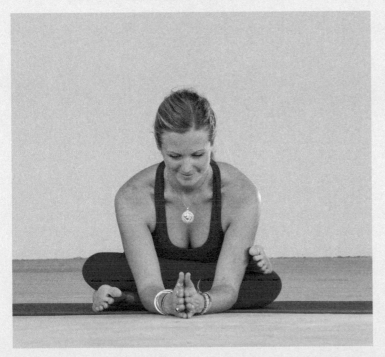

TIGHT HIPS Inhale to lengthen, exhale, and slowly fold forward to a comfortable level. Stay for 10 breaths and then repeat, with the left leg in front.

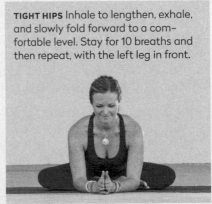

CHAPTER 3

Not all those who wander are lost

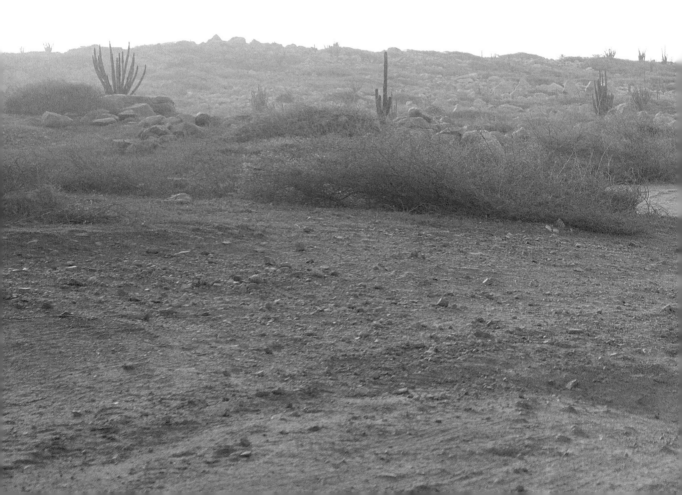

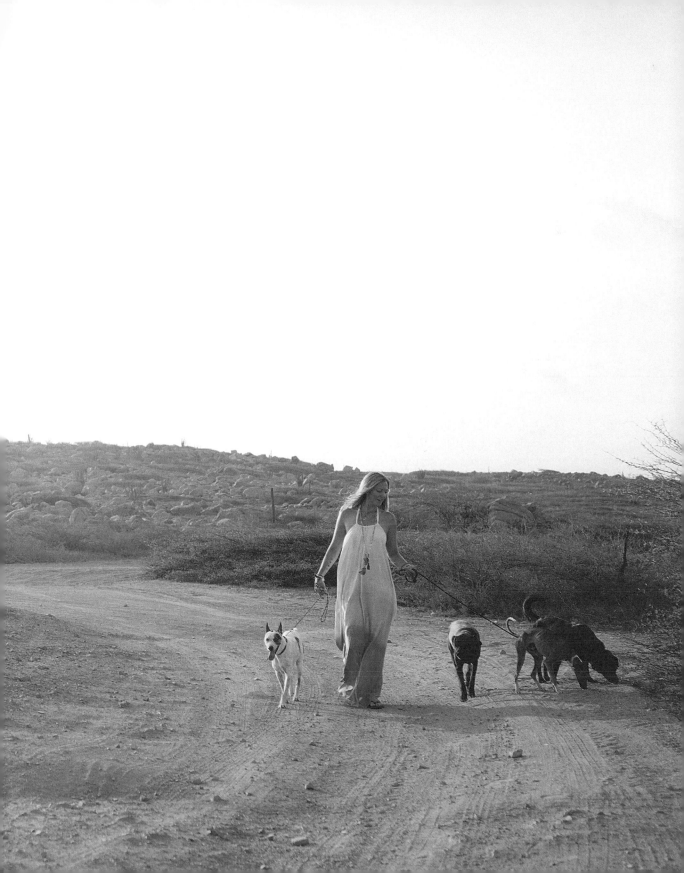

I didn't make a conscious decision to leave Sweden and not return, but when I bought a ticket to Costa Rica for the very first time, nineteen and anxious to see the world, my mom said to me with tears in her eyes, "I have a feeling you're never coming back." She was not exactly right, but she wasn't wrong either.

I knew I wanted to go somewhere far, far away and I knew I wanted to work on my Spanish, but I didn't know exactly where I wanted to go. I decided to take a big trip with two of my friends. At first we were going to Colombia but then changed our itinerary to Costa Rica at the very last second. The moment we landed, I felt I'd arrived someplace special, and even though we had planned to see many different parts of Central America, we ended up never leaving Costa Rica. After ten days of travel we made it down to Dominical, a small village that according to the guidebook was supposed to be "a laid-back surf town with a Snoop Dogg vibe." I fell in love right away—first with the place, then with a guy (of course). For the first time in my life I started to feel as if I belonged somewhere. This was my place to be. Slowly, one day at a time, I started changing. I took the meditation techniques I had learned at the meditation center in Sweden and started applying them to my life. I would wake up really early, before sunrise, and take a long walk on the beach. I'd find a beautiful spot to sit down and then would do my best to meditate. In the beginning it was hard; I'd have to keep reminding myself to focus on the breath. After a while it became really easy, like breathing. I would sit down and close my eyes, and meditation would just come. I didn't have to work for it. After a few weeks I was meditating mornings and evenings for at least thirty minutes each time, sometimes longer. I remember a friend of mine saying to me: "I saw you meditating on the beach and I needed to ask you something, but I didn't want to disturb you. After a while the spot you were sitting in filled up with people and children, but you didn't seem to notice. An hour later, when the sun set, it got really dark and the mosquitoes came out, but you were still sitting there."

I was in such a good space that meditation seemed entirely natural. I look back at those days of my life and can't help but smile. Life was so simple. I had no steady job and didn't have any money. I waitressed some days, bartended some days, and sometimes worked at a dive shop in between, but most of my time was spent on the beach,

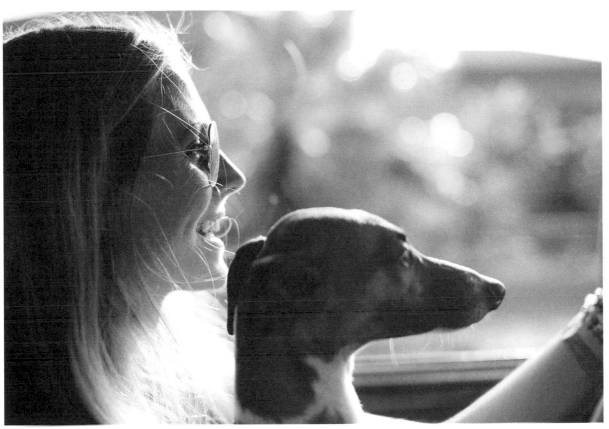

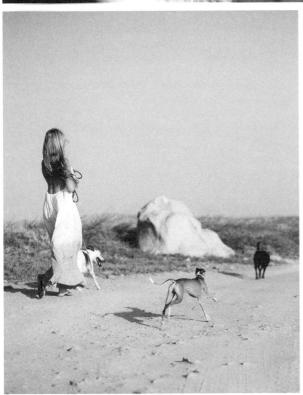

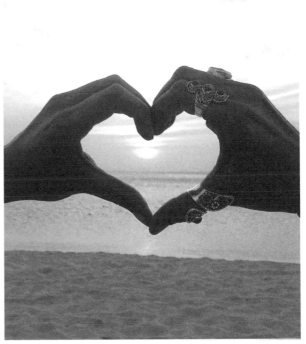

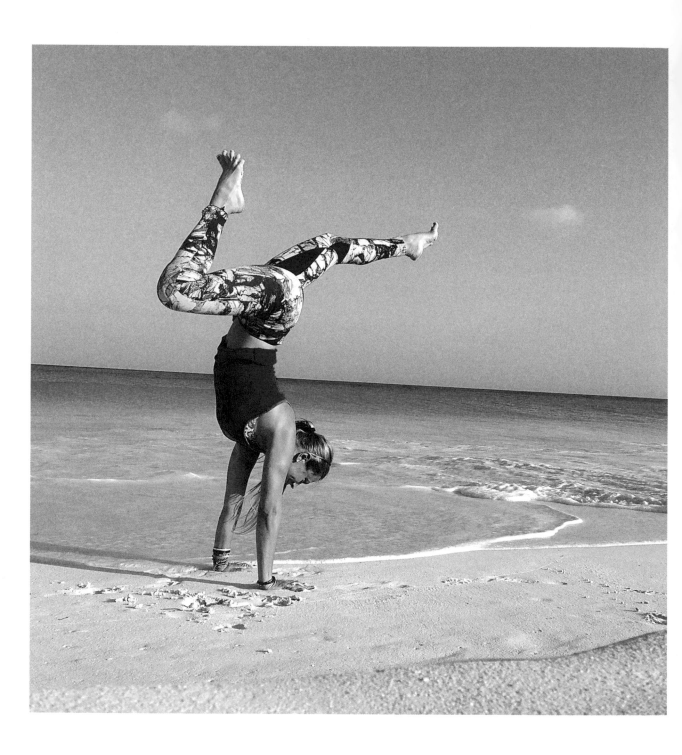

NOT ALL THOSE WHO WANDER ARE LOST

on my yoga mat, and in the surf. After a few months I went back to Sweden, packed up all of my belongings, and returned to Costa Rica on a one-way ticket, this time with a yoga mat strapped to my backpack.

I had been introduced to the practice of yoga during that one class I took in Thailand a few years earlier, but since I'd learned how to meditate, there was something pulling me strongly toward this five-thousand-year-old way of life that I couldn't quite understand. I took my first yoga class in Costa Rica with a teacher I'd met while hiking in the rain forest and I absolutely loved it. This type of yoga was very different from the class I'd taken in Thailand (or maybe I was the one who had changed and become different?). The presence I felt in the moment while slowly moving my body from pose to pose and the peace that filled me in Savasana at the end of class were different from anything I'd ever experienced before. I started going a few times a week to a small yoga studio in town. I practiced with several different teachers and tried different styles of yoga, but didn't get attached to a particular branch of yoga or a specific yoga teacher. I just loved moving my body together with my breath! For me it was meditation in movement. I started practicing every evening in the tiny shack I was renting on the beach. I'd roll out the mat on the kitchen floor, not really knowing if the poses I was doing were correct but simply doing what felt right. I could feel my body softening, and I spent many, many yoga sessions crying in hip- and heart openers. I had so much tension stuck in my body after years of not treating it right! Through yoga, I started unraveling the past, and little by little worked all the way to the center of my own heart—a place I hadn't been in touch with in many years. It didn't take long before I completely fell in love with yoga as a lifestyle and started looking forward to every moment spent on the mat.

I didn't need much and was happier than ever. Some mornings I'd wake up and have to decide who was going to have breakfast—me or Quila, a homeless puppy I'd adopted (she always won). It was okay. I ended up staying in Costa Rica for two and a half years, and it was during these years that I truly learned what happiness means. I had spent my whole life thinking I needed to fill my days with things to improve my "image." I had to look good, wear lots of makeup, buy nice clothes, be friends with the right people, have a skinny body, and so forth. As I peeled off the layers of who I had

"Do no harm, but take no shit."

become and started finding out who I truly was, I realized I didn't need any of those things. I didn't need a single object or situation to be happy. Happiness came from me, from my view of the world, not from external factors beyond my control. I stopped worrying so much about what everybody would think of me, and I started focusing more on what I was feeling inside. I knew that if I kept meditating, if I kept enjoying life, life would take me to the places I needed to be. I believed in this very simple philosophy so much that nothing seemed to bother me. If I trusted that things would work out in my favor, they always did.

For instance, after a year and a half of living in Costa Rica I started waitressing at a restaurant owned by a very unpleasant woman. I was now single, living on my own in a small shack on the beach, working with no goal in sight other than continuing to be very, very happy. The owner of the restaurant didn't like me from the second we met. She would make mean remarks, force me to work extra hours with no pay, and wouldn't let the chefs make me vegan food to eat (so I would work twelve-hour shifts with little or no food). I didn't mind. I knew her problems had absolutely nothing to do with me, but were merely a reflection of her own issues. So I continued working, making good friends with the rest of the staff, and enjoying the connections I formed with people traveling through town. The happier I was, the angrier she would get, and after I had worked at her restaurant for months, she kicked me out one day for showing up in a dark blue skirt instead of a black one (this was a low-key restaurant in a surfer town, and my only black skirt was in the wash). She yelled and cursed at me in front of the staff and told me to leave, as I was "embarrassing" the restaurant with my clothing. A little over the top, if you ask me! But I didn't get upset. In that moment I realized that there is a difference between going with the flow of life and seeing the good in everything that comes your way and letting people walk all over you. One of the mantras that I live by these days is: *Do no harm—but take no shit!*

The next morning I sat down on the beach at sunrise, meditated for a good hour, and decided that I'd had enough. I didn't want to work for that woman anymore. I was ready for something new, something different. Maybe something that paid me enough to cover my electricity bill (I had been living with candles lit at night for quite some time). But what could I do to change my situation, really? It was the off-season. Few people came through town during those months of the year because it rained every afternoon. I had no ticket out of the country, no money, nothing of significant material value. But not once did I doubt that I would receive an opportunity to create something different—I trusted in life's ability to care for me. Always! So I looked up at the sky from my meditation spot and said out loud: "Universe. I'm ready for something new. Bring it!"

That evening I went to work at the restaurant as usual. The owner came by my house to apologize (or actually to tell me they were understaffed and needed me to work, but I took it as an apology). I had no other way of making money at that moment, so I headed over. Halfway through my shift a big group of people came in to eat, eight or ten of them, and we immediately hit it off. I waited on their table and at one point overheard them talking about sustainable development and some kind of reforestation project. This was a subject that interested me greatly, so I joined the conversation, and at the end of the meal they asked me to sit down with them. I didn't care too much about keeping up appearances in front of the owner anymore, and since the restaurant was nearly empty, I sat down. Someone poured me a glass of wine, and we got to talking. It turned out they were all from a company that owned a lot of land in the mountains surrounding the area we were in, and they were in the process of building a luxury eco-resort, hoping to raise money to help the impoverished parts of the country. This all sounded extremely exciting to me—wealthy people on a mission, looking to improve the world. We spent a good hour talking, and after a little while the CEO asked me, "So, what about you? Are you happy here?" I thought about it and immediately answered, "No. I used to be happy here, but I decided just this morning I'm ready for something new."

He replied, "Why don't you come work for us? This might sound absolutely crazy and out of the blue, but so far we have only hired people that resonate with our hearts. We haven't seen a single résumé—we only want to work with people who have good energy and who are on the same path. Would you like to come onboard? We could really use someone to do assistant work for us, keep the team healthy, and handle travel and logistics."

"Are you kidding?" I asked. "No!" he said. Well . . . okay, then!

I walked into the restaurant office, took my apron off, and very dramatically threw it on the floor (I'd seen people do this in movies and it was something I always wanted to do) in front of the owner. "I quit!" I said. And I walked out. Two days later I was on a plane to Orange County, planning a meeting with executives to discuss million-dollar investments. I'm not kidding. This all happened, exactly the way I'm telling you. They gave me a big salary (highest I'd ever had before), I got to keep the team healthy, plan meals, and do general personal assistant work. It was also around this time that I started teaching yoga; I didn't have any formal yoga education, but I used my intuition and the knowledge I'd gathered from my own practice to teach gentle classes to the team in the mornings. It was wonderful!

Taking my first steps toward teaching yoga sparked something within me that I couldn't put my finger on, but it felt very, very important. It was years before I would make yoga my career, and I didn't know at the time how important these first classes would be. I'd fly back and forth between Costa Rica and California and Oregon with the company, and all of a sudden my life was very different. All I had to do was ask for it!

I remember sitting in a Porsche driving down the Pacific Coast Highway close to San Diego during the first trip I took with them, enjoying the breeze and the sunshine, and I realized: One week ago I couldn't pay my electricity bill and didn't have enough money to buy proper dog food. Now I'm here. This is how easy it is. If I want to change my life, I change my life. If I want abundance, I can create it. I am in charge.

These experiences changed my life and evolved into my very own life philosophy: We are all in charge of our own happiness. Life does not happen to us, it happens for us! By making ourselves victims of the situations around us, we start attracting experiences in which we'll always be victimized. By believing in the good of the universe and trusting in life's ability to take us where we need to go, we can create any type of living that we want. I had never cared at all about money or material things or any other type of "success" other than happiness. But I never knew how easily those things could be attracted, too! Happiness does not come from the outside. Allowing happiness to blossom from within attracts positive experiences. Trying to force things to happen,

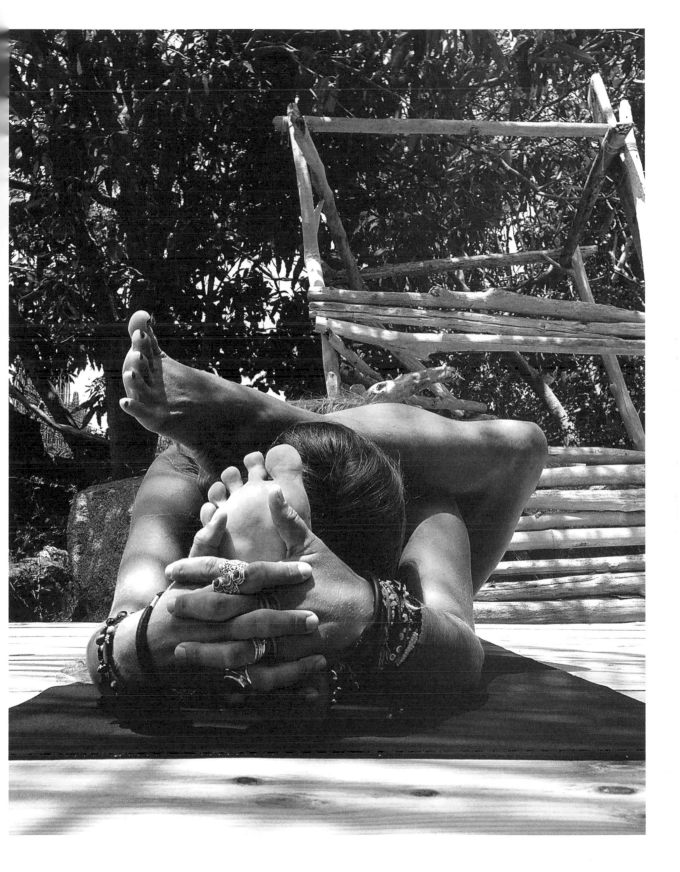

LOVING INSIGHTS

۶ Meditate, meditate, and keep on meditating until you've learned to let go of all the things you fear to lose.

۶ Take the step. Don't be afraid. Follow your intuition, wherever it takes you.

۶ You will always be okay! Money and material things come to you when you dare to trust in life's ability to take you exactly where you need to go. When we live in fear we create tense vibrations that keep the things we long for at a distance. Worrying is praying for what we don't want to happen. Focus on what you want, not what you fear!

۶ Do no harm—but take no shit!

۶ Ask the universe for what you want. If you don't know what you want in life, how are you ever going to create the life of your dreams? Write down everything you want to create. Be detailed. Take all the active steps you need to take. Ask for what you want and keep your intentions loving and clear.

۶ Explore the world and soak up the wisdom that lies in every lesson you learn along the way. Life is meant to be an adventure!

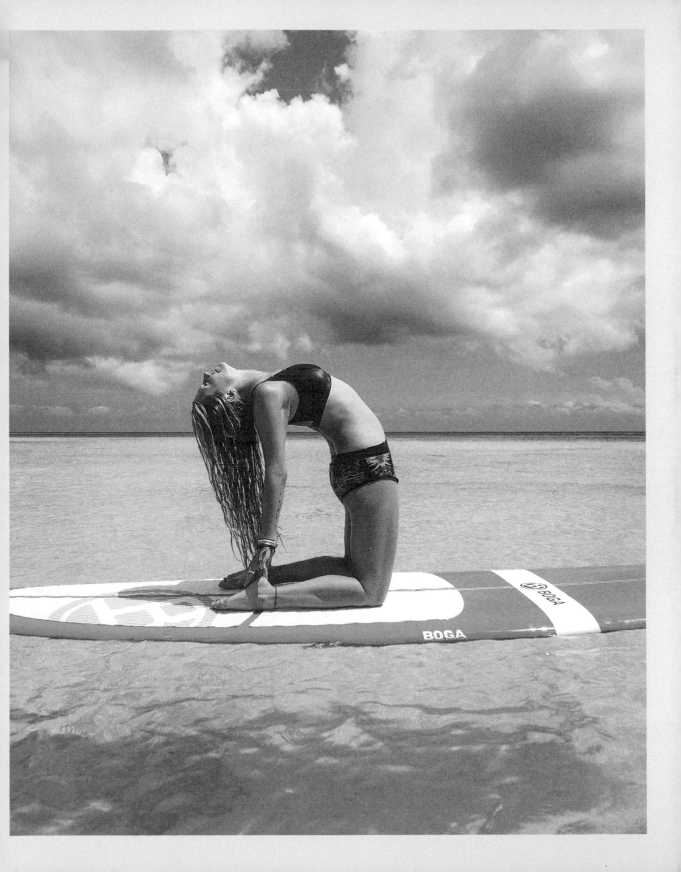

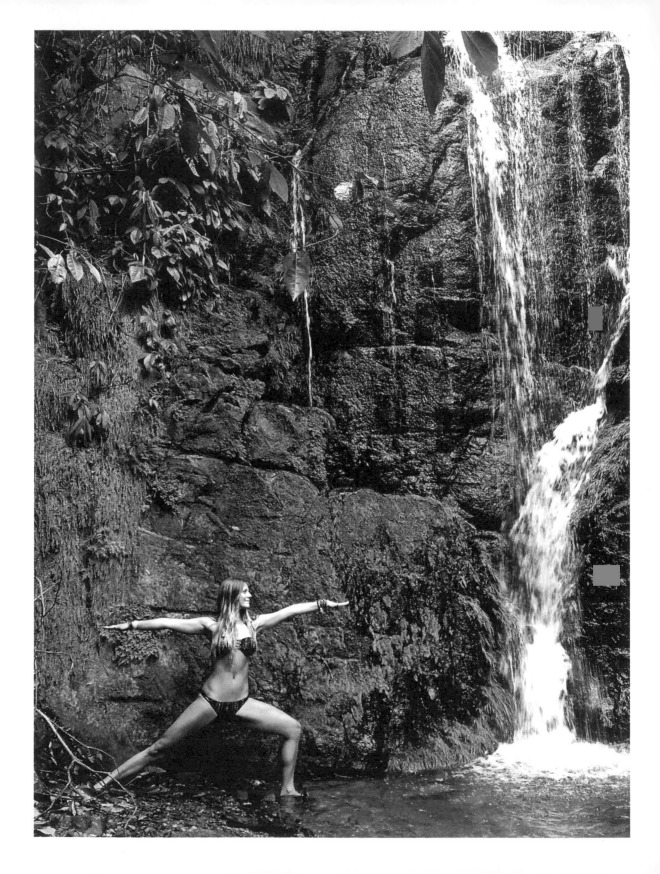

*"Opportunities are all around us—we just
have to believe in them to see them."*

---

judging how other people live their lives, or beating ourselves up about the past will never make us happy.

Opportunities are all around us—we just have to believe in them to see them.

A year or so later, I was starting to feel done with Costa Rica. I'd been there for almost three years, I'd learned a lot and made friends so close they had turned into family, but I felt deep inside that there was more left to explore in the world. I was living with my best friend in a small house with our dogs, I was still meditating daily, and I spent a lot of time in a commune in the mountains above our town. Here I learned about permaculture farming, and my yoga practice became stronger than it ever had been before. I met a shaman who told me my life's purpose; I traveled south for an ayahuasca ceremony that turned into one of the most intense spiritual experiences I had ever had. I meditated in caves, ate only raw food, and swam in waterfalls. Life was a whirlwind and it was beautiful. But after three years in the country I had the same feeling I'd had a year earlier: I was ready for the next big experience. I left the company I was working for, on good terms, and used the money I had made to travel.

After a little time on my own in California and eventually in Portland, Oregon, I went to Sweden to spend Christmas with my family. I still had my house and my things (and my dog of course!) in Costa Rica, and my intention was to go back there right after Christmas to figure out what I wanted to do for the next year. In Sweden my dad said to me: "I want to take your little sister on a vacation in March. Why don't you come with us?"

"I don't know," I said. I had already been in Sweden for a full month and was itching to get back to Dominical.

"I would love to spend some time with you. How about we all go some place close to Costa Rica so your flight back won't be so expensive?"

"Sure!" I said. "That could work. So where do you want to go?"

"There is a new direct flight from Stockholm to Aruba. How does that sound? Come have two weeks of vacation with us, and then go to Costa Rica from there."

"Aruba?" I said. "Where is that?" ❦

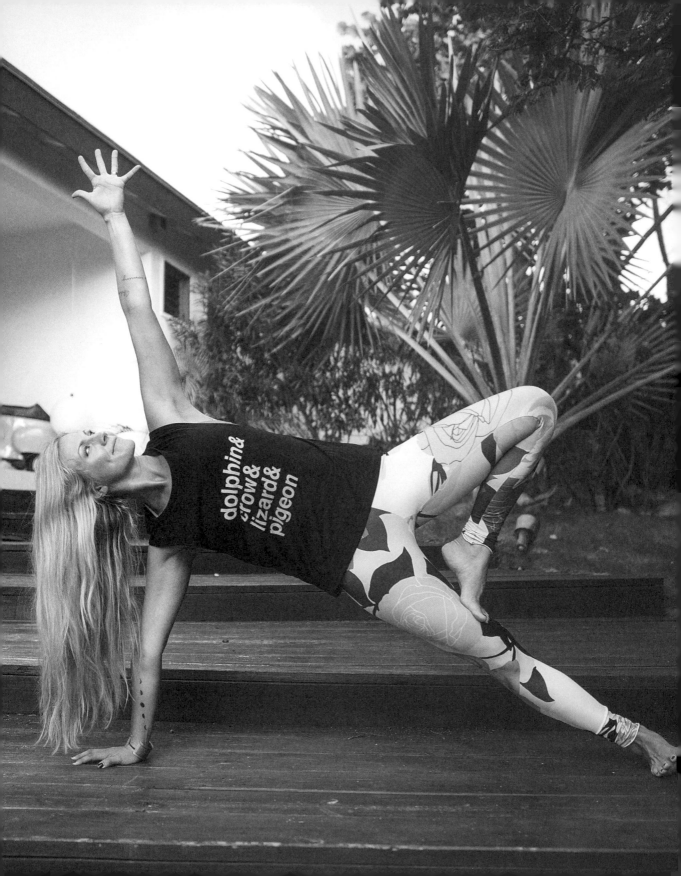

GUACAMOLE

½ yellow onion ✤ 4 cloves garlic ✤ 2 big ripe avocados ✤ Juice of half a lemon ✤ Salt ✤ Pepper

Put finely chopped garlic and onion in a medium-sized bowl. Add the avocados and squeeze in lemon juice to taste. Mash together (I love to use a potato masher!) and season with salt and pepper. Eat right away (guacamole is meant to be eaten on the spot, standing over the kitchen counter).

I make this guacamole every week. I like it with a lot of garlic and I don't use tomatoes as in traditional recipes because I like it thick and chunky. If you're eating your guac with chips, remember the chips can already be quite salty, so don't go too crazy with the salt! If you set the avocado pits in the guacamole it will last a little bit longer.

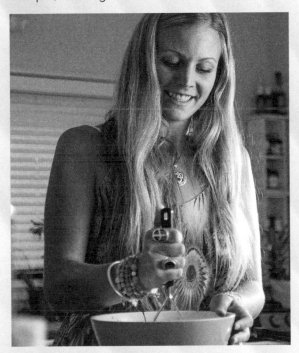

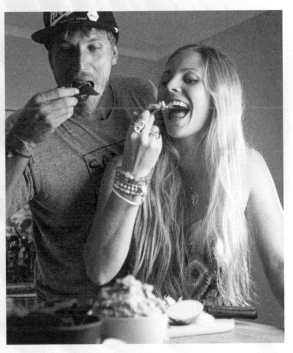

HEAVENLY HUMMUS

½ cup tahini (sesame paste) ✤ Juice of one big lemon ✤ 1 (15-ounce) can chickpeas ✤ 2 tablespoons olive oil ✤ 1 clove garlic ✤ Sea salt ✤ Cayenne pepper

Pour tahini and lemon juice in a food processor or a high-speed blender and mix until smooth. Add chickpeas, olive oil, and garlic and blend well. You might have to stop the blender a few times to stir, making sure it doesn't stick. Add sea salt and a dash of cayenne pepper. If you like your hummus even smoother, add a few tablespoons of water.

I love hummus because it can be served with almost anything! I love to eat my hummus with vegetables as a dip, but it's also great with a salad or on a sandwich. A good food processor will make this recipe easier, but a blender will work well, too. If you want to take your hummus to the next level, remove the peel from each chickpea . . . and it will become even smoother!

Core, Balance, and Shoulder Work

Good core strength is important for the practice of yoga, as well as for our well-being as a whole. Your abdominals support your lower back, the spine, and the internal organs. If you suffer from lower back pain, chances are you need to strengthen the core to help support the lumbar area of the spine. Our core is also where our sense of confidence lies, the base for how we walk through life.

The exercises in this chapter can be done as part of a full yoga session or separately on their own. Think about engaging the belly and pulling the lower ribs in toward the spine to connect to the transverse abdominals.

The neck and shoulders are where we tend to hold a lot of stress and tension, and if you spend lots of time sitting in front of the computer, these exercises will be great for you. You can even do them at your desk at the office! Sit on the edge of a chair, keeping your spine long and a yoga strap or a belt close by to use if you need it.

I love that the things we do in our yoga practice truly help us create better posture even off the yoga mat. "Draw the shoulders down the back" or "Lengthen the spine," common yoga cues, work just as well when you're stuck in traffic or standing in line at the grocery store.

We need balance in all parts of our lives, and the yoga mat is a great place to start cultivating that! Plant your feet firmly on the ground so that you can grow tall without losing your balance in life.

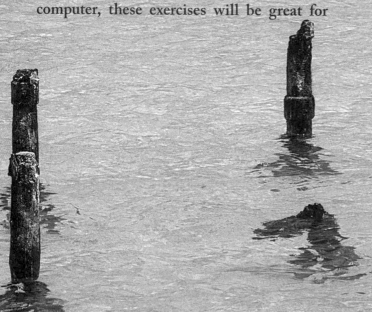

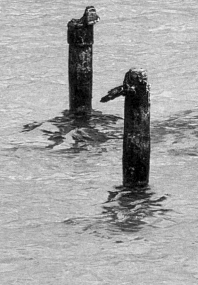

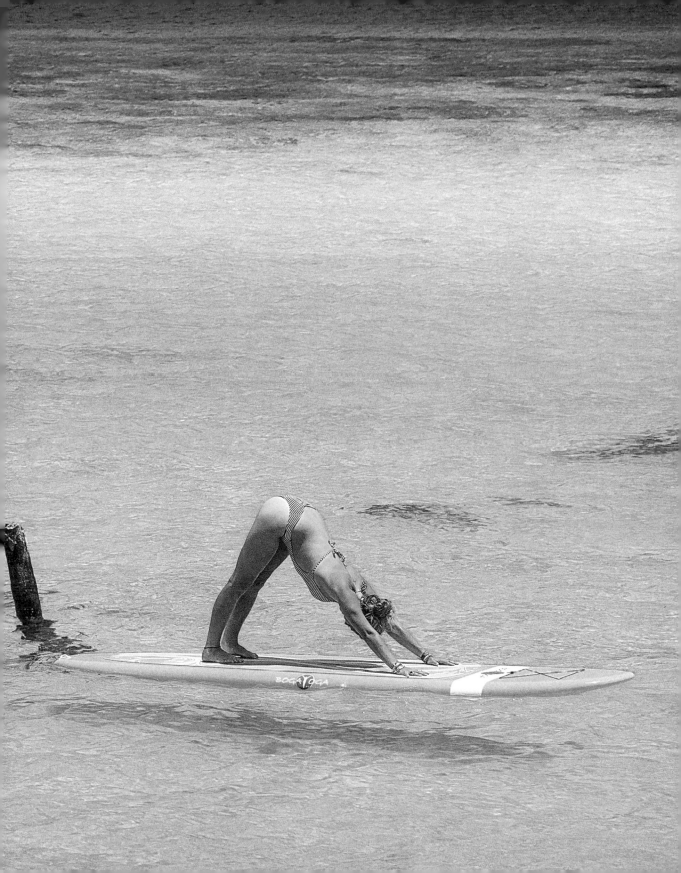

LEG LIFTS

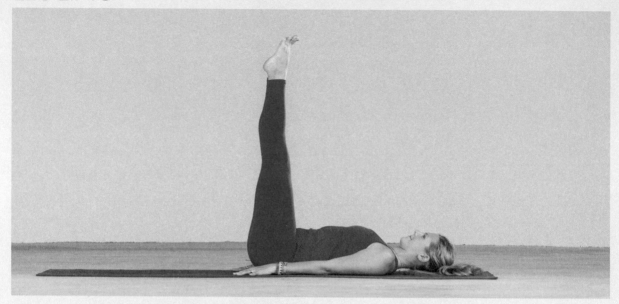

1 Lie down. Extend both legs straight up toward the sky so that the ankles line up with the hips. Press the balls of the feet up toward the sky and spread your toes (we call this "flointing" the feet!); this will help engage the inner thighs and activate the legs. Connect the two big toes together and keep your arms down by your sides. Inhale here.

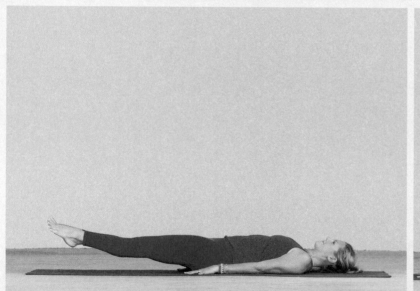
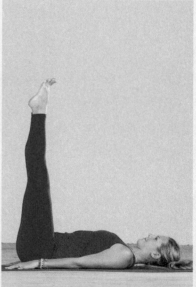

2 Exhale and lower the legs until they're hovering right above the ground. Keep the two big toes together the entire time and make sure that the back of the head and the shoulders are still resting on the mat. Engage your core!

3 Inhale and lift the legs back up. Repeat as many times as you can while still keeping the breath steady (try 20!), always moving with the flow of the inhales and exhales.

NAVASANA AND ARDHA NAVASANA / BOAT POSE AND HALF BOAT POSE

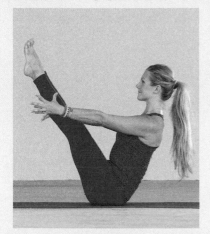

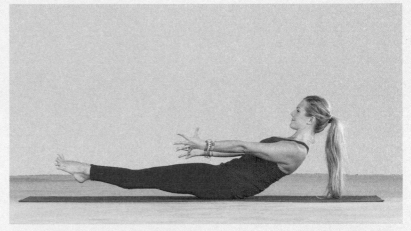

1 Come into a seated position with the soles of the feet touching the floor. Walk the toes in toward the sit bones as much as you can, and then lift both legs, extending them up and hugging to the midline while engaging the inner thighs. Shift your weight toward the front of the sit bones, away from the tailbone, and keep the spine long while lifting from the heart. Make sure you're not rounding the lower back!

2 Lower the body from Navasana to Ardha Navasana. Keep the lower edge of the shoulder blades lifted off the floor and let the legs hover above the mat. Keep the arms reaching forward and activate the core by pulling the lower ribs in toward the center line of the body. Exhale and make your way back to Navasana. Inhale and lower to Ardha Navasana. Exhale and come back to Navasana. Repeat together with the breath 5 to 10 times or as many times as you can without lifting from or rounding the lower back.

NAVASANA, VARIATION

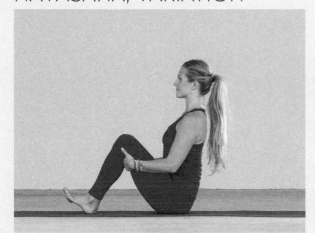

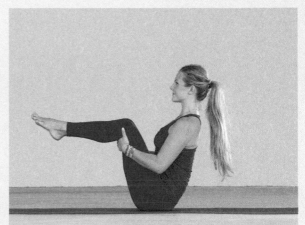

1 If you are just beginning to learn this pose and are still working on building core strength, you can choose to keep the heels on the mat, staying in this position for a few breaths while lengthening the spine. Even though you're not moving, you want to feel your core working for you!

2 If you have tight hamstrings or if you find it difficult to move into Navasana with straight legs, do this variation with the shins parallel to the mat. Inhale to lower, exhale to come back up with your knees bent.

CORE EXERCISE: EAGLE VARIATION

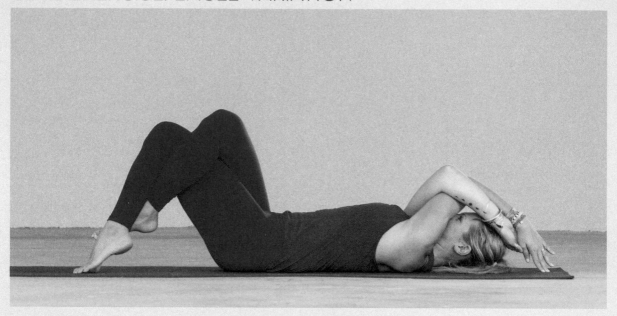

1 Lie down. Cross the right leg over the left, hooking the right foot around the left ankle. Extend your arms out to the sides, perpendicular to the body, and then cross the left elbow over the right in front of you. You can either press the

backs of the hands together here, or bring the palms all the way together. Keep the toes pressing into the mat, inhale, and reach your arms over your head until your fingertips can touch the mat above you.

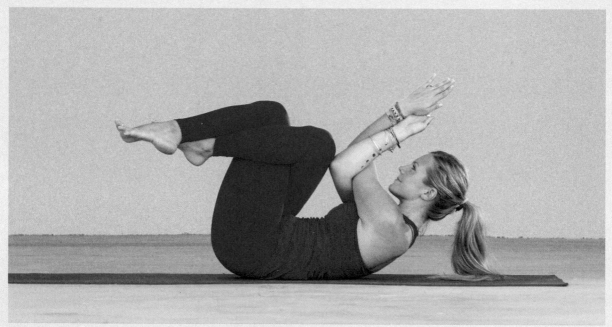

2 Exhale and lift the legs and arms off the mat so that your knees and elbows connect, pulling the navel into the spine, feeling the abdominals engage. Inhale to lower,

touching the fingertips and the toes to the mat. Exhale to connect elbows and knees. Repeat 10 times and then switch sides with both arms and legs to do the other side.

CORE, BALANCE, AND SHOULDER WORK

SEATED NECK STRETCH

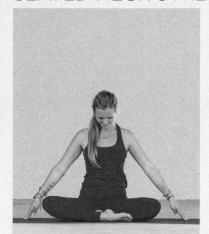

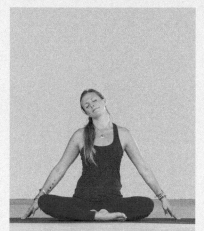

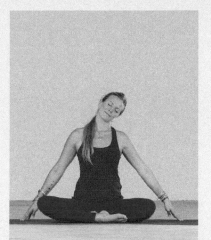

1 Come into a comfortable seated position. If you have a sensitive lower back, place a folded blanket beneath your sit bones. Sit up tall and extend your arms out to the sides, keeping your fingertips connected to the floor. Walk the fingers as far away from the hips as you can without letting them lift off the ground. Drop your head down and gaze toward your feet, keeping your chin to your chest.

2 Gently tilt your head toward the right so that the right ear draws toward the right shoulder. Move your head slowly, keeping a slight tuck of the chin. Breathe deeply.

3 Bring your chin to your chest again and then gently move your head to the left. Use the breath to draw some space into the parts of your neck that feel tight. Move your head left to right, right to left, without tilting your head back.

Dress comfortably when you practice yoga. I usually wear leggings or yoga pants with a tighter tank top and a loose off-the-shoulder shirt on top. That way I can remove a layer when I start sweating and nothing will droop over my head in Downward-Facing Dog. At the end of a class I usually feel a little chilly, and then I have a layer to put on top again.

The most important part is that you feel comfortable and that you can move freely. Remember that big seams or zippers are too bulky for positions in which you are lying down, so try to find a pair of leggings that aren't too embellished. If you sweat a whole lot or practice hot yoga (yoga in a heated room), sweat-wicking performance materials are great (high-functioning yoga pants can even make arm balances easier when we're sweating!). If you're practicing a gentler style of yoga in which you're not sweating that much, natural materials like cotton and bamboo feel amazing. Do you practice yoga at home? Give it a try in your birthday suit! Practicing naked is extremely liberating. Love your body. Think about all that it does for you every day.

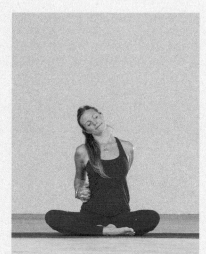

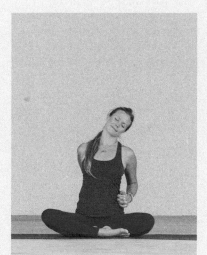

4 Come back to center. Interlace your fingers behind your back and extend the arms behind you, pressing the palms of the hands together. Move your hands as far to the right side of the torso as you can, squeezing the right elbow inward. Relax your shoulders and then softly drop your head to the right. Take a few moments here, breathing into the sensation of the neck.

5 Do the same thing on the other side. Inhale to extend the arms straight back behind you, interlacing the fingers with the opposite thumb on top. Then move the knuckles as far over to the left as you can and gently tilt your head to the left. Take a few deep breaths here and then come back to center.

SEATED SHOULDER STRETCH

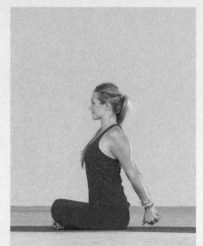

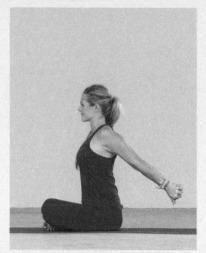

TIGHT HIPS If your hips and shoulders are tight, you can use a strap and a block to help you.

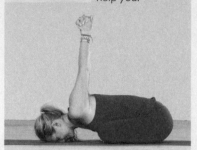

1 In a seated position with legs crossed, interlace your fingers behind you. Extend the arms straight back behind you while keeping the spine long.

2 Lift the arms as high off the floor as you can while keeping the shoulders drawn down away from the ears.

3 Engage your core and fold forward. If you can, rest your forehead on the mat and keep pressing the knuckles toward the back of your head. Stay for 5 breaths and then come back up. Switch legs so the opposite leg is to the front and then interlace the fingers with the opposite thumb on top and fold forward again.

GARUDASANA / SEATED EAGLE

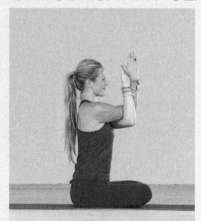

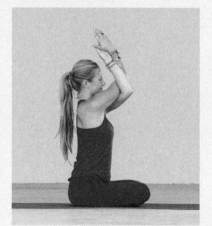

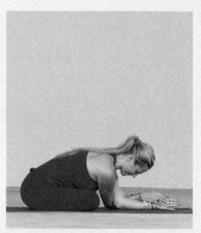

1 In a seated position, inhale to extend the arms straight out to the sides. Exhale and give yourself a big hug, crossing the right elbow over the left. Then place either the backs of the hands together or the palms of the hands together if you have the space. With your hands at the center of your face, relax your shoulders and keep the spine long.

2 Inhale and lift your elbows up, reaching the fingertips higher toward the sky.

3 Exhale and fold forward. Inhale and come back up. Repeat 5 times and then fold forward and take a few breaths here. Create space in the upper midback and breathe deeply into the shoulders. When you're ready, come back up and repeat with the left arm crossed over the right and the opposite leg in front.

GOMUKHASANA ARMS

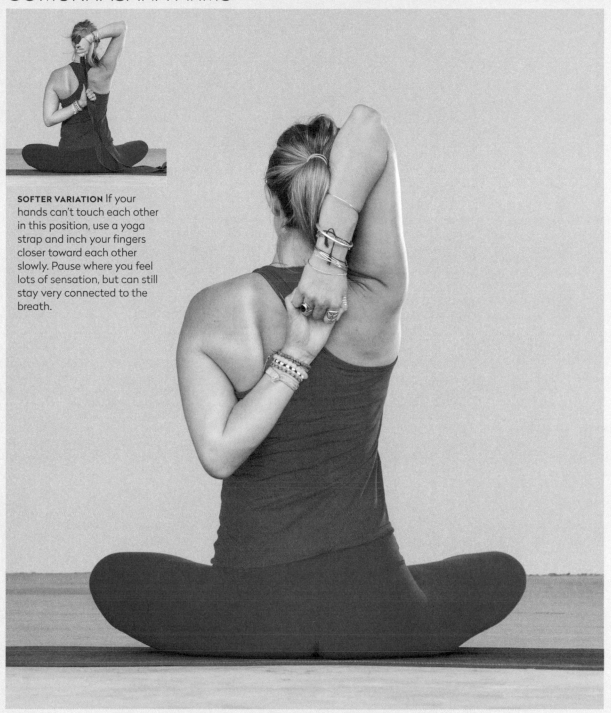

SOFTER VARIATION If your hands can't touch each other in this position, use a yoga strap and inch your fingers closer toward each other slowly. Pause where you feel lots of sensation, but can still stay very connected to the breath.

Reach the right arm straight up toward the sky and let the left arm come from below. Bend the elbows and start reaching your fingertips toward each other until your hands meet, if possible. Try to keep one elbow pointing upward and the other one pointing down. Stay for 5 to 10 breaths and then switch arms.

VRKSASANA / TREE POSE

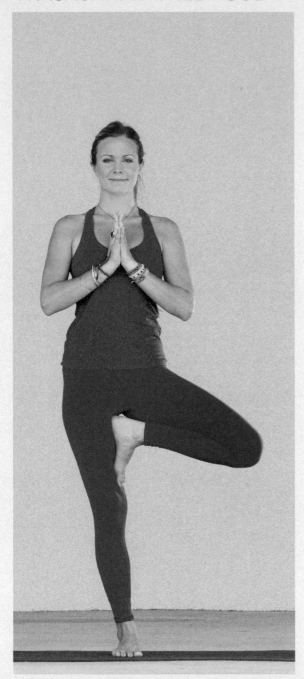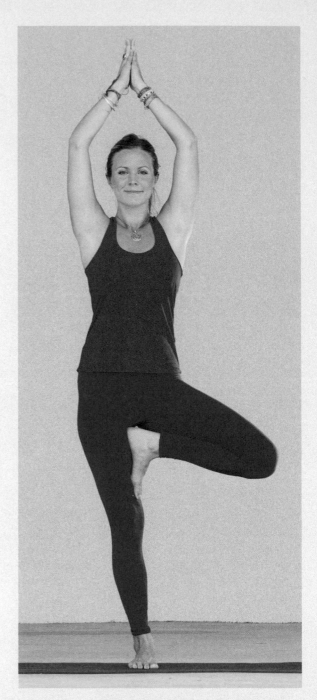

Come into a standing position. Move your weight to the right foot and lift the left leg off the ground, placing the left heel toward the inner right thigh. Reach your arms up and bring the palms together. Let the left knee point outward but keep drawing the frontal point of the left hip forward. Find your balance here for 10 breaths and then switch sides.

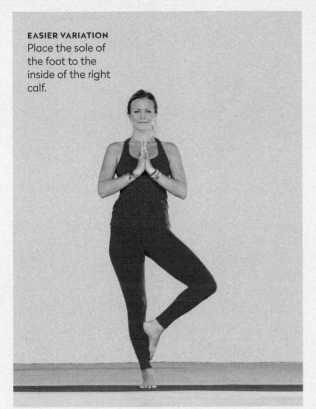

EASIER VARIATION
Place the sole of the foot to the inside of the right calf.

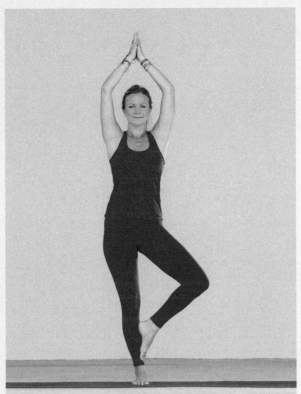

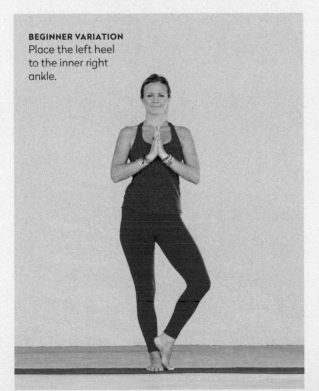

BEGINNER VARIATION
Place the left heel to the inner right ankle.

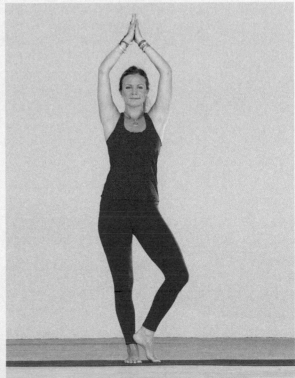

UTTHITA HASTA PADANGUSTHASANA/
EXTENDED BIG TOE POSE

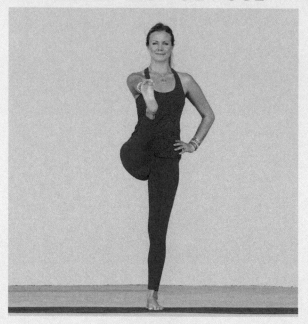

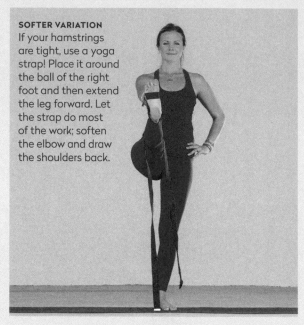

SOFTER VARIATION
If your hamstrings are tight, use a yoga strap! Place it around the ball of the right foot and then extend the leg forward. Let the strap do most of the work; soften the elbow and draw the shoulders back.

1 Come into a standing position. Shift your weight over to the left foot and bring the right knee into the chest. Use your peace sign fingers (index and middle finger) to hook

around the right big toe, and then gently extend the right leg straight out in front of you. Pull the right hip down so it stays level with the left, and engage the inner thigh.

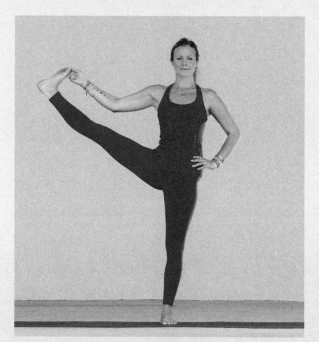

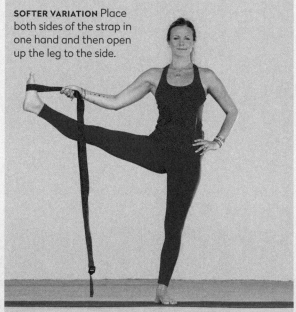

SOFTER VARIATION Place both sides of the strap in one hand and then open up the leg to the side.

2 Extend the leg out to the side and do your best to keep your hips neutral with the front of the hipbones pointing forward.

72

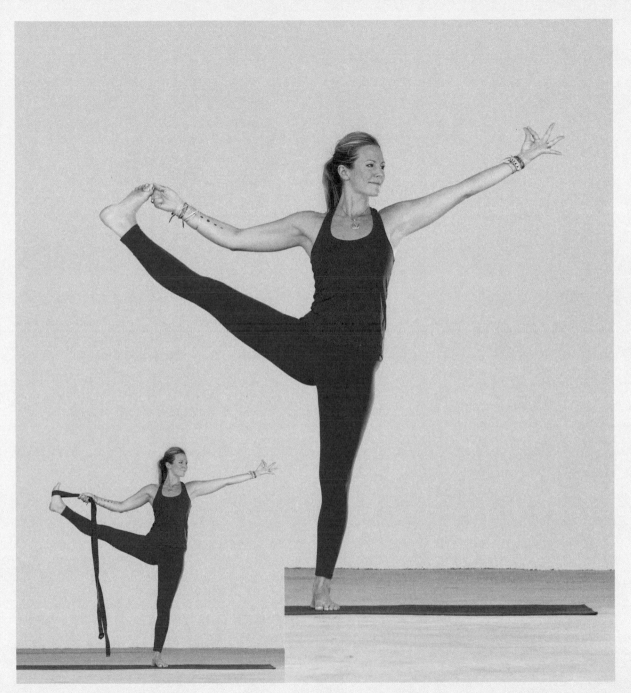

3 Gaze to the left to challenge your
balance further.

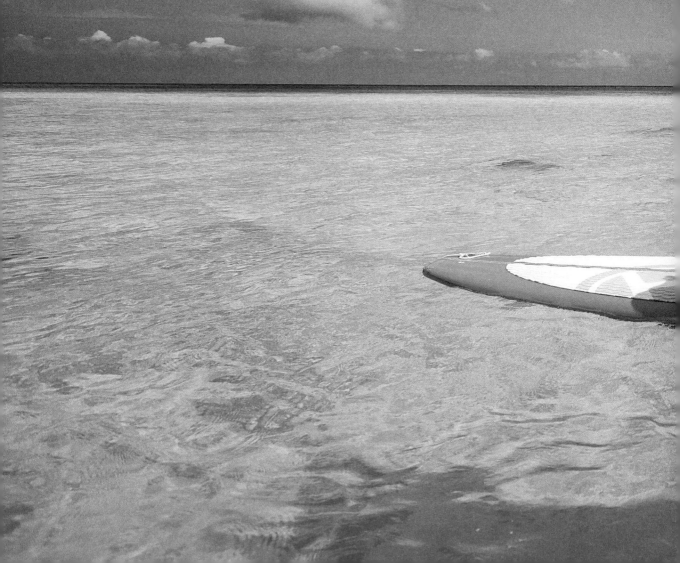

CHAPTER 4

The body is a place for the soul to reside in

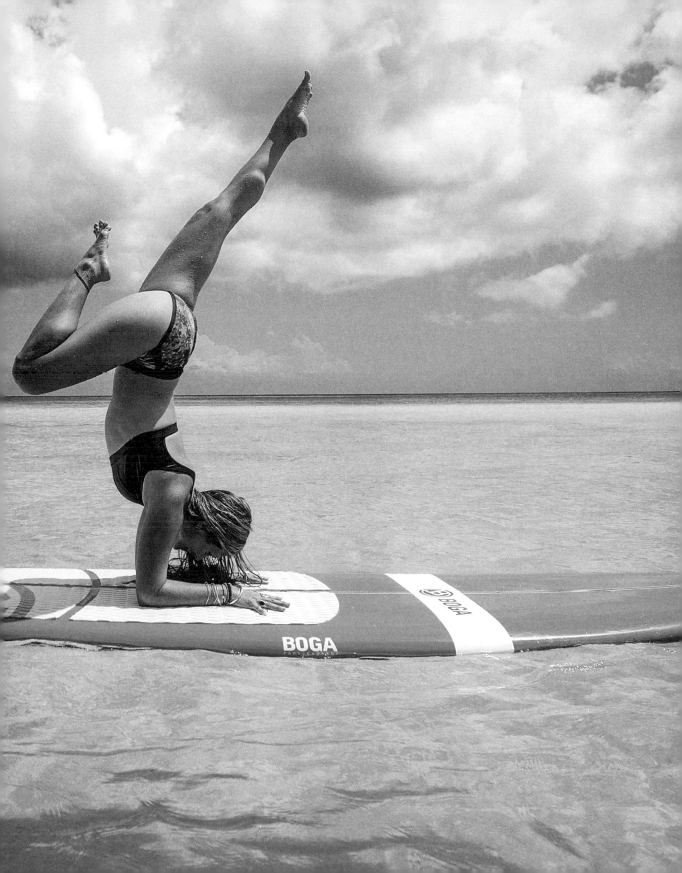

I flew to Aruba from Sweden together with my family, planning to spend two weeks there before heading back home to Costa Rica. I had never been to Aruba before and was mesmerized by the beauty of this small Caribbean island.

On my very first day there I went to meditate on the beach at sunset, and walking along the shore I decided it would be nice if I could rent a surfboard and maybe see if there was a good spot to surf in the waters around the island. I asked some random guy on the beach, and he told me there was a surf shop downtown.

The next day I made my way there. I got a cab, found the shop, opened the door, and bumped straight into a very tall, blond, handsome guy in board shorts. "Hi," he said. I wanted to say "Hi" back, but for some reason the words got stuck in the back of my throat—I couldn't talk! I felt my face turn red. *What was happening? Could I be nervous about talking to some guy I'd never met before?* This was very unusual for me. I normally never get nervous, and especially not around surfer dudes. Who was this man? I found out his name was Dennis and that he was Aruban and also the manager of the shop. I spent almost an hour in there wanting to talk to him but feeling very awkward about it. There was something special, even nerve-racking about this guy that I couldn't pinpoint. In the end I left the shop, went back to the hotel, and decided that it would have been a stupid idea anyway; what would be the point of getting to know someone living in Aruba? I never planned to come back here.

For one full week following that day, I woke up every single morning thinking about this guy Dennis. I couldn't understand it. I barely knew his name! After a week I finally summoned all of my courage and headed back to the shop. It was closed. The next day I tried again. I had never fought to get any man's attention before; all of the relationships I'd been in so far had just kind of happened on their own. Pursuing a guy, on a tiny island in the Caribbean that I'd never visited before, was very out of my comfort zone. This time the shop was open, but he wasn't there. Again I was nervous and I didn't want to ask his friends about him, so I lingered as long as I could, buying all sorts of things I didn't actually need.

Finally he appeared. He casually said hello but didn't come up to talk to me (probably because I was blushing and focusing all of my attention on a small spot on the floor), and again I was unable to speak. I couldn't figure out what the hell was wrong

THE BODY IS A PLACE FOR THE SOUL TO RESIDE IN

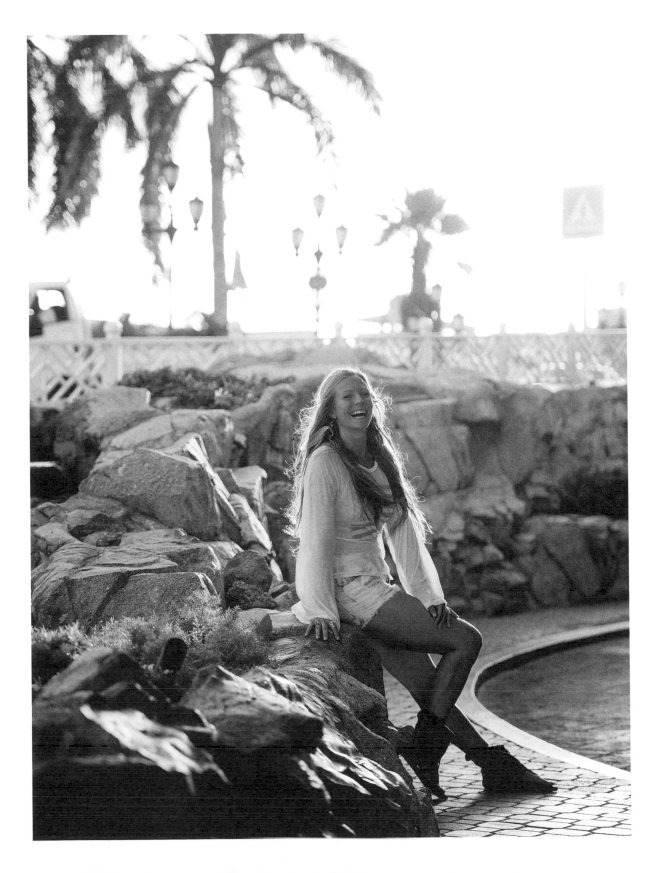

with me, so I quickly paid for my things and left. Walking across the open-air mall I suddenly felt someone watching me, so I turned around and there he was. He was leaning out of the shop, hanging on to the doorframe, with messy hair and a curious look on his face. I took a deep breath, flashed him a *huge* smile, and kept walking.

He came running after me. "Hey! I get off in twenty minutes and I was going to go catch some waves. I know we don't really know each other, but do you want to come?"

"Yes," I said. "I do."

Four and a half years later I said, "I do," to a whole different kind of question, but this time in front of our friends and family, barefoot, wearing a white dress. Dennis's hair is still messy and he still has that curious look on his face most of the time, and we now live together on the north coast of Aruba with our dogs. It's been quite the ride getting here! After spending only five days with Dennis while I was in Aruba on vacation, I went back to Costa Rica, where my best friend immediately told me I needed to return to Aruba. I had found the love of my life and everyone around me could tell! Before I knew it I was on a plane to start the rest of my life with someone I had known for just a few days. When you know, you know!

Moving to a new country, leaving my house, changing my life, was actually the easiest thing in the world. I'd never felt this comfortable with any other person, and it was clear from the start that we were simply meant to be with each other. We moved in together on the very first day and have been living side by side ever since.

It was here in Aruba that I found stability for the first time in my life. I no longer felt the intense urge to travel and to keep moving from place to place. With Dennis I felt at home. It was also here, around this time, that I started making the transition toward becoming a full-time yoga teacher.

I didn't have a job or a work permit in Aruba, and I knew I didn't want to work in the evenings anymore. I didn't want to waitress or have small jobs here and there: I wanted to find something substantial and make it my own. All I could think of was: *I want to teach yoga*. I'd taught yoga to the people in the company I worked for the year before, and also a little here and there to friends, but I'd never made it anything official. Now here in Aruba with my whole life a blank page in front of me, I thought:

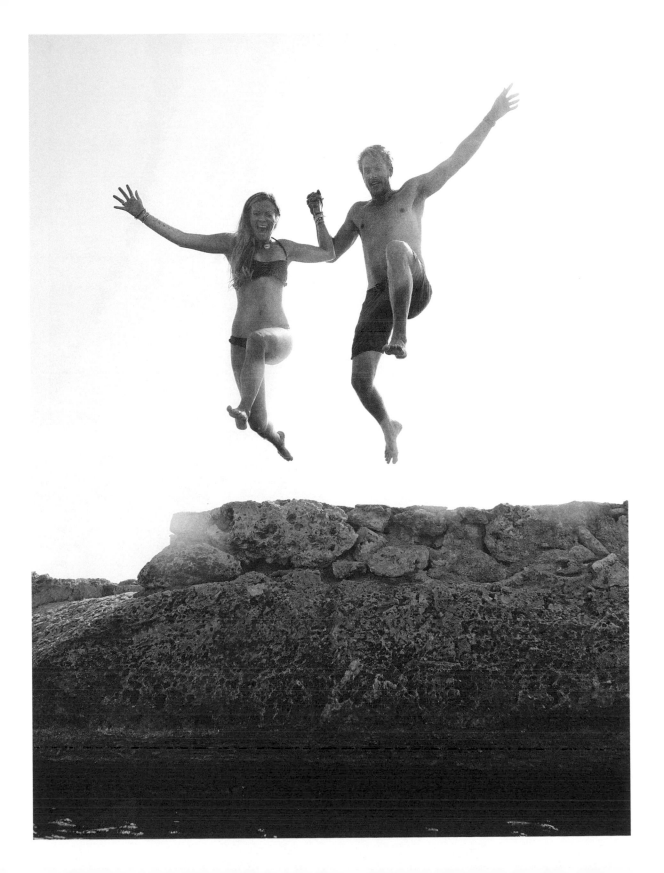

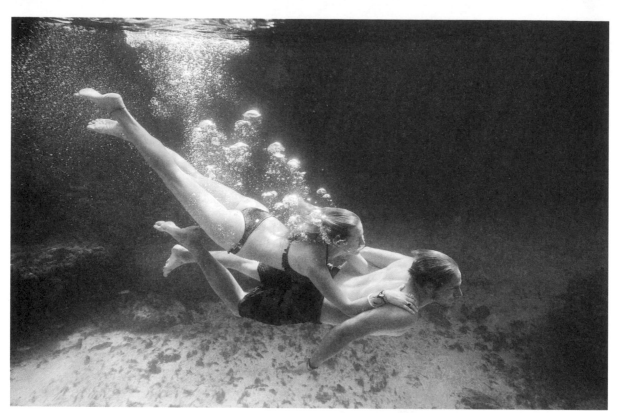

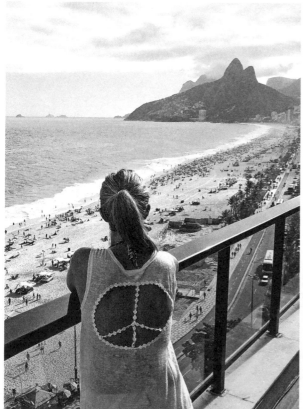

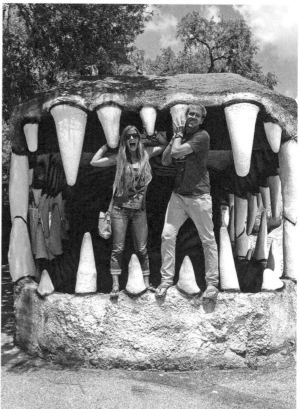

"A good body is every body."

_____

I can make this happen! I am in charge of my happiness. What kind of life do I want? There was no substantial yoga community on the island, and I found my way to a lady who was giving lessons in her house. I started helping her with her classes and managing her small studio, and I realized quickly that there was a huge potential for yoga to grow on the island.

I started studying and reading every book about yoga I could get my hands on, and during this period my practice grew from spiritual to very physical. My meditation practice had always been there; normally people find their way to the physical aspect of yoga first and meditation and spirituality second, but I started the other way around. I was very comfortable meditating and working with different breathing techniques, but because of the back pain I had suffered from since my early teens I had never dared to move into a very physical practice. I was born with scoliosis and an elevated hip, and a car accident and a white-water rafting accident had left my spine a mess. I'd been fearful to try advanced asanas (poses) or to move too quickly, but after my first few years of very gentle practice I felt I was ready to move forward.

I started practicing yoga at our house every single day but with another goal in addition to centering my thoughts: to sweat. I'd come to the mat and move in every way my body wanted to move, and instead of shying away from the poses that caused my back to act up, I tried to stay in them a little longer. I learned how to walk the fine line between embracing the intensity of a pose and overdoing it. I started building some serious core strength. One of the reasons I'd had such a bad back my whole life was that I had very little core strength to support it! I had always avoided strong, dynamic exercises, thinking they would aggravate my pain, when in fact they were what I needed the most. The key is to be very patient with your body and take it one step at a time. If I had thrown myself immediately into a dynamic practice, I probably would have ended up with more pain than ever before. But I listened to what my body was telling me every step of the way, and I also let my breath guide my body instead of the other way around. This principle is key in my teaching to this day.

I summoned up the courage to begin teaching a yoga class of my own, on the beach in front of a hotel. We were in the sand on beach towels, under a small grape tree, and if I had three or four people in my class I would call Dennis afterward, giddy with

LOVING INSIGHTS

☙ Set your roots. Build your foundation and let the adventures you have ahead of you grow from a place of stability.

☙ Be patient with your body!

☙ Even if you can't see how your dream is going to come true, focus on the idea of it happening. You don't need to know every step ahead of you to be able to move forward.

☙ Don't get stuck with labels! Eat what keeps your body and soul happy.

☙ You are perfect the way you already are. Thinking we will be happier by changing our bodies is simply scratching at the surface. What lies beneath? What do you really need to be happy?

☙ Concentrate on what your body does for you, not what it looks like.

☙ Focusing on the things you perceive as flaws only magnifies them. See your own beauty.

☙ Eat well and exercise for the right reasons. Love your body first, change it (if needed) later.

☙ Health and happiness are important. Not what your ass looks like in a pair of jeans!

☙ Love your body. Love your soul.

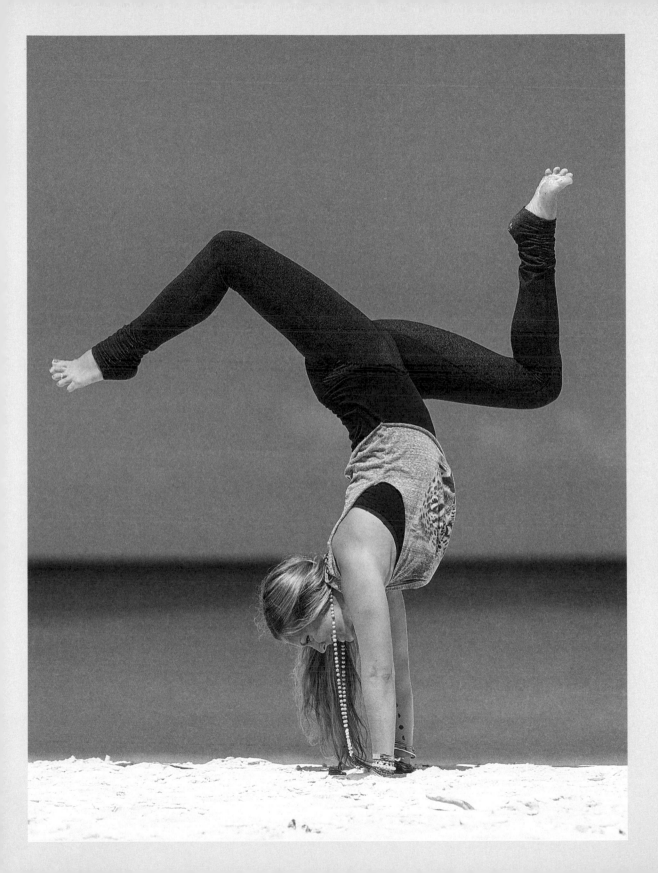

excitement. "Four people came to my class!!!!" I would scream into the phone. "Four people! To *my* class!"

Every night I would work on my sequences, trying to write things down so that I wouldn't be so nervous about teaching, but failing miserably every time. I cannot prepare a class. It's impossible. Even now, if I try to prepare what I'm going to teach, I always end up throwing everything out the window the second I see the class and create my flow on the spot. The people in class are the ones teaching me everything I need to know about what to do. It's impossible to prepare when I don't know who is going to attend and what their energy levels will be.

But I tried hard during my first days of teaching and would always end up driving to class in the morning with a knot in my stomach—I was so nervous! But the class always went well, the words came easily to me, and I loved guiding people through extra-long Savasanas. One day the owner of the hotel I had my classes in front of came to participate. "I've been hearing about these classes of yours," he said. "I hear you're good!" Apparently word was getting around about my classes and had reached all the way to the owner, who lived in the United States.

After class he invited me to breakfast, and before I knew it, I was hired by the hotel to teach yoga on a regular basis as an in-house yoga instructor. I booked my first teacher training that very day. If I was really going to pursue this, I needed to make sure I had all the credentials. I completed my first 200 hours of teacher training sessions feeling very confident. I had already been teaching for a while, and everything I knew about sequencing and anatomy I had learned on my own. My real studies since then have come from workshops, training sessions, and practice with amazing teachers all over the world and from immersing myself in the world of yoga. And from my students, of course!

The yoga community on the island started to grow. I added classes and invited teachers from abroad to come lead retreats at the resort. Fast-forward two years, and I was teaching twenty-four classes a week, mostly Vinyasa-based classes but also meditation, restorative yoga, and SUP yoga, which is yoga classes on stand-up paddleboards on the ocean. Classes were big and I was working my butt off to evolve as a teacher.

All the while I was working hard on my own mat. Through a mix of restorative yoga

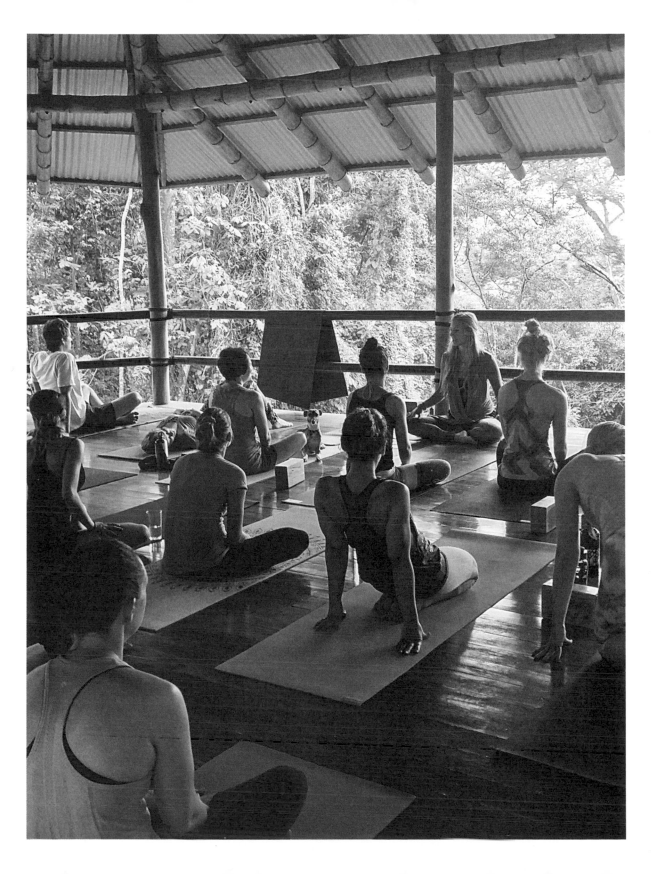

to heal and create flexibility and a dynamic practice to build strength, my back was feeling great. I had built a lot of muscle tone and was even getting the hang of inversions. Handstands, headstands, forearm stands, and advanced poses I never in my wildest dreams thought would be a part of my practice started coming my way with ease. I took the dogs for long walks in between classes (by now we had three), went for runs on the beach, and continued practicing strong, dynamic vinyasa every day. I was feeling great, but the more I moved my body the more I started realizing: I was getting really hungry!

I absolutely love food and I love to cook (and eat!), but since my first year living in Costa Rica I had been a very strict vegan. This lifestyle makes me feel the healthiest, and to this day what I aim for in my day-to-day life, but I've learned to let go of the label. I was a strict vegan for six years, staying far, far away from anything that contained even the possibility of animal products. When I say I was strict, I mean strict— I wouldn't cook in a pan if it might have been used to cook anything with dairy or meat in it, no matter how many times it'd been cleaned. I had a roommate who would stash cans of tuna under her bed because I didn't allow any animal products in the house. Really, I was super vegan!

Also, I liked to share my views on veganism with the world. Loudly. Talking about the health hazards of eating meat and the ethics behind slaughtering animals is not great dinner conversation, I'll tell you that. Labeling yourself as one thing or another puts you in a box that's very hard to get yourself out of. As I got more and more into teaching yoga, with all the exercise I was doing and all the classes I was teaching, I felt I needed something more. If I lived in a place that had a farmer's market or a health-food store, I probably would have kept the label of being vegan, but it was not easy being vegan in Aruba.

Now the situation has improved slightly, but at the time, there were no vegetarian restaurants, no health-food stores, no farmer's markets—nothing! I found myself obsessing over keeping up with my vegan eating habits. Preparing dinner became a struggle. I even got annoyed walking through the grocery store, feeling like there was nothing proper for me to eat. I fought Dennis about it, feeling as though I had found a big flaw in our lives on the island.

It took me a little while to understand that I needed to transition toward a more vegetarian diet. It was hard in the beginning because I was very attached to the vegan label I had given myself. With time, however, I started eating some cheese and then some yogurt and then even a little ice cream. Becoming more relaxed about my eating habits helped me stay fueled throughout the day without feeling stressed about what I was putting into my body. A little bit of ice cream is not going to ruin your life. Guilt, however, could!

I realized that being healthy and caring for your body is all about mind-set. By obsessing over every little thing I was putting in my body, I had created a harsh, judgmental environment for myself. A tense environment doesn't allow us to create the happiness we need; to have a happy, healthy body we need to think happy, healthy thoughts about it! Loving your body means loving every part of it, not just when it suits your mind or when you've created the "perfect" conditions for it.

It's not that difficult to love our bodies when we're working out a lot, following a strict regimen, eating a specific diet—when we fit ourselves into a mold that society has told us we need to fit into. But this love is not whole or true. It's the mind tricking us into believing we're happy because we are trying to control the body. The second you "fall off the wagon," the moment you eat that dessert or skip a workout or whatever else you've decided is essential for you to be happy about the way your body looks, you will feel guilty.

Why is it so important to be thin? Fit? Muscular? Why is it that we on some level feel that we are not good enough the way we are? Who taught us that we need to see a certain number on a scale to be happy? When was it decided that we need to look a certain way to feel happy about who we are? Yes, we want to be healthy. Yes, we want to feel good. But the world we live in is full of unrealistic expectations that absolutely no one can live up to. We all have different ideas about what it means to have a good body, but my definition is this: A good body is every body. Your body, the way it is now in this moment, is a good body. You have legs to walk you through the world, a mouth to speak with, a heart to feel, hands for touching. Your body is a miracle just the way it is. *You* are a miracle just the way you are. Start treating yourself that way, and exercise and healthy eating habits will come easily. Stop judging yourself! When we truly love who we are, we will naturally want to care for our bodies. It's where our soul resides. We need to stop comparing ourselves to others and start loving ourselves just the way we are. Of course we have a hard time finding an exercise or diet routine to stick to—the

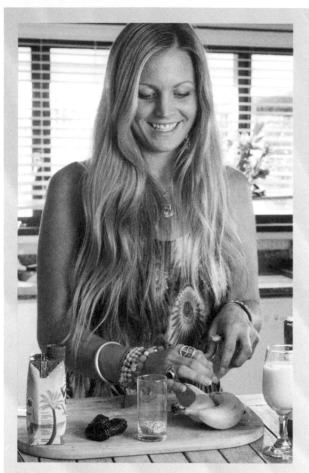

RAW BANANA ICE CREAM

2 bananas, peeled, chopped and frozen ❧
1 tablespoon maple syrup ❧ 1 teaspoon organic
vanilla bean powder ❧ 2 tablespoons chopped
almonds

Peel the bananas, cut them in pieces, and put in an airtight container in the freezer for at least 12 hours. When you feel a craving for ice cream coming on, simply place the frozen bananas in a blender, add the maple syrup and the vanilla powder, and get blending! In the beginning, the bananas will spin around the blender, but when they start to melt they will turn into a perfect, amazingly delicious soft-serve ice cream! Garnish with chopped almonds and serve right away. You can also flavor the "ice cream" with pretty much anything you want: cacao, almond butter, berries, fresh mint. The sky's the limit!

RAW VEGAN BOUNTY BLISS

1 (13.5-ounce) can of organic coconut milk ❧
½ cup melted coconut oil ❧ 2 cups raw cacao
powder ❧ Pinch Himalayan salt ❧ ½ cup
unsweetened shredded coconut ❧ 8 tablespoons
maple syrup

To make the coconut cream, place the can of coconut milk in the fridge overnight or at least for a few hours. When you open the can, a thick layer of "cream" will have gathered at the very top of the can, and the water will have sunk to the bottom. You want to use all of this cream!

   Mix coconut oil, cacao powder, Himalayan salt, 5 tablespoons of the maple syrup, and the coconut cream in a bowl and stir until smooth. Pour half of the chocolate mixture in a pan and put in the freezer for ten minutes. Meanwhile, mix shredded coconut with the remaining maple syrup until it becomes a thick paste. Take the pan out of the freezer and spread the coconut mixture on top. Pour the rest of the chocolate mixture into the pan. Put the mixture back in the freezer for 30 minutes, then cut in pieces and enjoy!

The more coconut cream you use, the more your chocolate will resemble milk chocolate. Instead of shredded coconut you can use any filling you want (how about almond butter?), and you can add nuts, raisins, goji berries, or anything you feel like to the chocolate. Another tip is to flavor the chocolate with a few drops of peppermint oil. Since the chocolate is made from coconut oil it will melt fairly quickly, so don't leave it out for too long!

THE BODY IS A PLACE FOR THE SOUL TO RESIDE IN

whole reason we feel we need one is that deep down we feel we are not good enough as we are.

Telling yourself you're not good enough is not loving yourself. Looking in the mirror and seeing only flaws is not loving yourself. Exercising or dieting simply because you want to change your body is not loving yourself. And I don't in any way mean that exercising is not good for you—quite the opposite. It's the way we look at ourselves that we need to change. The most difficult thing is not to find an exercise or diet routine that we can stick to, but to deeply accept that we are already okay. You are okay. You are more than okay! You are beautiful just the way you are.

I say, change it up! Instead of thinking you need to change your body so you can love your body ("after I've lost twenty pounds, I'll be happy with who I am"), do it the other way around. Love your body so you can change it. If we keep exercising in order to change because we are not already perfect, that exercise is always going to be negative and to have a negative effect on all aspects of our being—mind, body, soul. You think staring at yourself in the mirror, jaws clenched, while running on the treadmill is good for your body? Think again. You think taking away the joy of eating delicious food is good for your body?

Think again.

We are energetic beings. What you send out, you get back. If you don't want your entire life to revolve around the shape of your physical body (which in the big scheme of things is so insignificant!), you need to realize this and make fundamental changes from the inside instead. Yoga is good. It can also be done wrong, sure—practicing without mindfulness can definitely be compared to running on the treadmill, jaws clenched. Are you in your body on the mat? Or in your mind? Do you feel the moment? Or are you focused on nailing that next pose, getting to the next step? Our minds can turn anything into ego. Which is why again we need to come back to a place of love.

The good thing about yoga is that it is so accepting, so loving, we can all do it, no matter our age or body type. We can practice whether we're tired or energized, during the day or night . . . as long as the breath is there. Daily yoga helps because the thing that hurts us in the long run is our mind, not our body. We can weigh a million pounds, but that alone is not going to make us unhappy. It's our mind's perception of this fact that will make us unhappy. It's the thinking that hurts us. When we say "I should" or "they shouldn't" or "I would be better if . . ."—this is the reason we feel so inadequate. Yoga helps calm the mind so we can free ourselves from these destructive thought patterns.

I used to think I wasn't good enough, thin enough, smart enough, pretty enough. And I was always trying to find something that would help me get better, thinner, smarter, prettier, because then at last I would be happy. But I finally realized that nothing from the outside will ever fix my inside. Even if I am a supermodel or the smartest person in the world, my mind will keep trying to find the next thing to fix. That is why we have to find balance and happiness inside, not outside. Exercise is good and taking care of our body is good, but we need to do it mindfully. Once we realize that we are already beautiful, intelligent, perfect, the rest will fall into place.

We will start making decisions throughout our day that will heal our body. And we will make these decisions automatically, because we love ourselves. So it will be natural to go for the fruit instead of candy, to move, to meditate, to eat meals that build us up instead of eating things that break us down. And this is where balance comes from.

It took me a long time to find a balance in life, and I still struggle through days when all I want to do is lie in bed and eat my weight in chocolate. Who doesn't? And sometimes I do that too, trust me—and it's okay! As long as those days are not overpowering your life. Find what makes you happy, accept your highs and lows, and remember: this too shall pass. Stay beautiful, inside and out. Love your body. Love your soul.

These days I stay away from labels completely. I eat a diet that consists of mostly whole foods, vegetables and fruits, grains, and legumes. I also eat pasta, bread, cheese, chocolate, ice cream . . . you name it. I know that the problem is not the foods I put in my body, but the way I think about my body. When I focus on loving who I am, I naturally go for foods that do me good. I no longer have to label myself *vegan* or *vegetarian* to feel happy about my diet—I just need to feel content! I know that eating an abundance of healthy whole nonprocessed foods make me feel balanced and happy, so I strive for that, but it doesn't mean I can't have dessert. I sometimes joke that dessert is the whole point of eating dinner! And I mean it. Life is meant to be enjoyed. Don't cut yourself off from the sweet things in life. Just listen to your body and you'll know just how much sweetness you need. As with everything, balance is key. ✸

Use daily affirmations to attract all of the beautiful things you want in life. Affirmations are positive statements about ourselves or our situation that can help us reprogram how we think, feel, and perceive our surroundings. An affirmation will enforce your belief in what you're looking to manifest and create in your life. If you're looking to de-stress, for example, instead of thinking "I want to get rid of stress" or "I want to find peace," affirm: "I am calm." Imagining your desired state of being as something that already exists here and now will transform life in a very powerful way. Here are some beautiful affirmations to use for your day-to-day life:

"I am a magnet for the goodness of life. I attract beautiful experiences, qualities, and situations. Love, peace, abundance, and joy are coming my way. All good things flow to me, and I receive freely without hesitation. I am free. I am blessed. I am whole. I am one with all that is."

"I am STRONG. I have the power to turn any challenging situation to my favor. Negativity bounces off me, as I choose to invite only love into my world. If fear does enter my life, I will use my inner strength to transform it into loving power. I am strong, and I know that every challenge I'm presented with in life is a loving reminder from the universe to connect back to my inner power. I do not hesitate to use my strength when needed."

SO HAM
"I AM"

I like to repeat this to myself when meditating w/ each inspiration + expiration

Vinyasa and Heart Openers

Vinyasa means flow, or a gradual movement that takes you from one point and allows you to land in the next. Vinyasa is sometimes described as breath-synchronized movement, meaning movement and breath united as one. The word *vinyasa* is now used in yoga classes to describe the connection between poses and can also be used as a collection of movements, as the ones showed in this chapter. You'll recognize the vinyasa as part of the Sun Salutation from chapter one. A vinyasa, as a noun, is usually practiced repeatedly in styles of yoga such as Ashtanga and Vinyasa Flow. The vinyasa strengthens the body, opens the heart, and creates and maintains heat when we're practicing on the mat.

It's extremely important that you learn how to practice the vinyasa correctly and that you have good posture! Since we repeat the vinyasa so often in class, you could injure yourself if you practice a pose like Chaturanga incorrectly. Listen to your body and adapt the poses when you need to so that you find a variation that's perfect for you.

Backbends, or heart openers, do exactly that: they open the heart. Physically and emotionally. When you open up the back of the heart and across the chest, you create space for the heart, which is both valuable and liberating! When you are practicing backbends, you must try to distribute the space as evenly as you can throughout the spine, and focus on the right part of the back. The lumbar area of the spine, the lower back, is usually very flexible, and we generally need more strength here than space. The same goes for the neck. Try to focus your backbends around the part of the spine that needs the most opening: the very back of the heart, the thoracic spine. That's why it's called a heart opener—we actually open up right at the center of the heart.

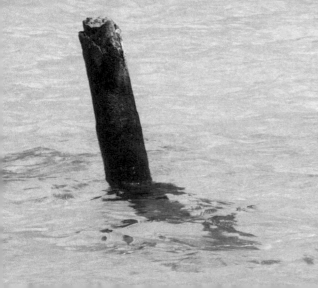

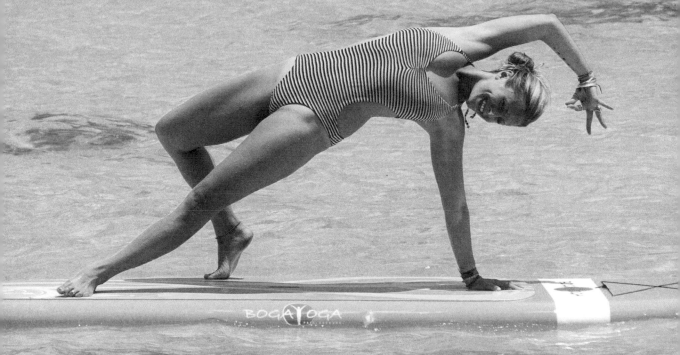

VINYASA

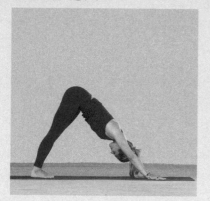
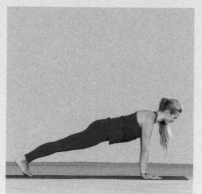
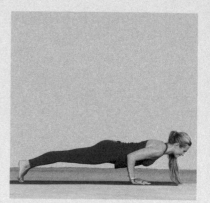

1 Come into tabletop position with your hands placed shoulder distance apart. Line the shoulders up with the wrists and the hips with the knees. Tuck your toes under and send your hips up and back, coming into Downward-Facing Dog. Adjust the space between your hands and feet if needed. With your feet hip distance apart, widen through the sit bones and draw the heels toward the earth. Press the thumbs and index fingers down, grounding through the inner wrist, and wrap the triceps back. Relax the neck and engage the inner thighs.

2 From Downward-Facing Dog, shift your weight forward and make your way into Plank Pose. Line the shoulders up with the wrists, draw your lower ribs in toward the body, and elongate the tailbone toward the heels. Actively press the earth away from you so you're not sinking into the shoulders. Press the heels to the back of the mat and let the chest draw you forward. Activate both your core and your legs.

3 Take a deep breath in and shift your weight slightly farther forward, over the wrists. Exhale and bend your elbows to Chaturanga Dandasana. Here you want the shoulders to line up with the elbows and the elbows to line up with the wrists. Keep the thumbs pressing to the ground, the ribs drawing inward, and the legs strong. Even though it's a tricky pose to stay in, relax your face and neck!

VINYASA FOR BEGINNERS

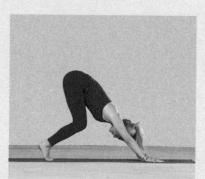
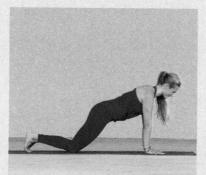
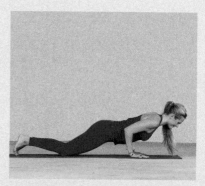

1 Come to tabletop position with your hands and knees on the floor. Tuck your toes and lift your hips up and back while keeping your knees bent. Let your heels come high off the ground and let your chest press toward the top of your thighs, lengthening the lower back. Wrap the triceps back and relax your neck.

2 Float your body forward to Plank Pose with the shoulders lining up with the wrists, and then bring the knees down to the earth.

3 With your knees still on the ground, slightly shift your weight forward and bend your elbows, coming into a half Chaturanga with your knees on the floor. Find the 90-degree angle of the shoulders, elbows, and wrists. Engage your core.

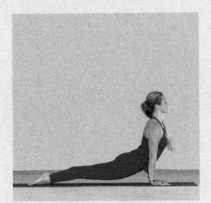

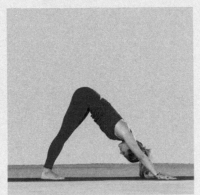

4 Inhale and actively press your toes to the back of the mat, lifting your heart into Upward-Facing Dog. Press the tops of the feet onto the mat and lift your thighs off the floor. Think of the crown of your head as an extension of your spine and lift your gaze without tilting your head all the way back. Keep the heart open, widening through the collarbones!

5 Tuck your toes, engage your core, and pull your hips up and back to Downward-Facing Dog.

Besides a yoga mat, a few other props can be very useful when you're practicing yoga. I personally use straps, blocks, and blankets in my own home practice. Think about these props as support that you can use when you need it; they are not crutches or in any way a sign of your not being good enough. Props can help you better your alignment and also deepen certain poses in a safe way. Using blocks in the right places means that you're smart and focusing on good posture, not that you're too stiff to reach the floor. I encourage all my students to use blocks whenever needed.

Yoga straps work great as an elongation of your arms when you're working the shoulders or hamstrings or are in standing balances. Blankets are great to use folded up under your hips for meditation, or to keep your body warm at the end of practice.

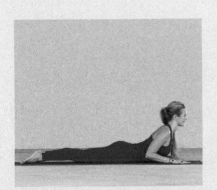

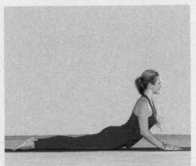

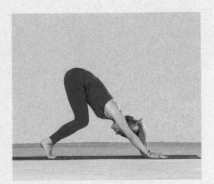

4 Come all the way down to the mat and place your hands slightly in front of your shoulders.

5 Press the palms to the mat and lift your chest off the floor, coming into Cobra Pose. Find a comfortable distance between your chest and the yoga mat, where you feel the upper back engaged and no pain in the lower back.

6 Tuck your toes under and move through to a tabletop position and back to Downward-Facing Dog.

VINYASA AND HEART OPENERS

CAMATKARASANA / WILD THING

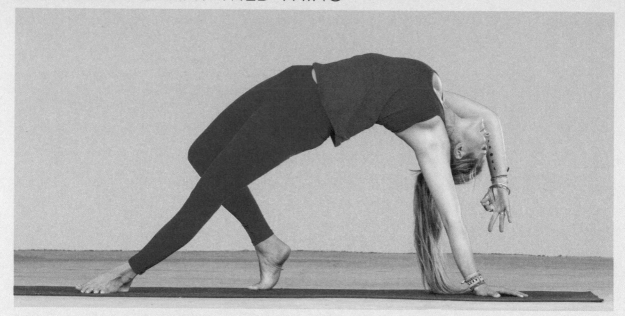

Make your way to Downward-Facing Dog. Inhale and extend the right leg up and back behind you. Bend the knee and open up through the hip. Let the right foot become heavy and gently flip your dog over, landing with the ball of the foot right behind the left knee on the mat. Feel the feet grounded to the earth, lift up through the hips, open the heart, and let your head hang back. Breathe deeply and enjoy this beautiful heart opener! Engage your core to come back to Three-Legged Downward-Facing Dog, lower the foot, and then do the other side.

SETU BANDHA SARVANGASANA / BRIDGE POSE

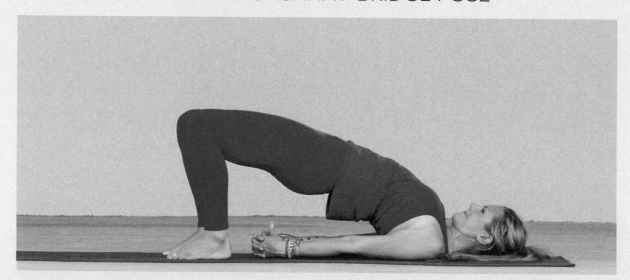

Lie down with your feet grounded on the earth, hip distance apart. Find a neutral place for the lower back, press the two big toes down, and inhale to lift the hips up. Bring the hips as high as you can without having to squeeze or overactivate the glutes. Interlace the fingers beneath you; wiggle the forearms and the elbows together and create more space for the back of the heart by grounding the arms. Let the head stay still, keeping the gaze up the entire time. Engage the inner thighs and make sure the knees stay in line with the ankles without tilting out to the sides. Stay for 5 slow breaths and then release the hands and gently come down.

URDHVA DHANURASANA / WHEEL POSE

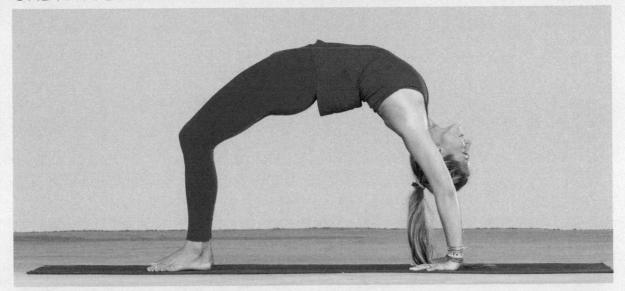

Begin in Bridge Pose with the arms resting down by your sides. Reach your arms straight up toward the sky, plugging the arms into the sockets of the shoulders. Ground the shoulders to the mat and reverse the palms of the hands on either side of the ears, shoulder distance apart. Press your hands down and lift up. Pause lightly on the crown of your head and squeeze your elbows inwards toward one another; press your chest toward your elbows, then lift all the way up into Wheel. Keep a very slight tuck of the chin, relax the neck, and fully engage the legs! Stay for five breaths. To release the pose, tuck your chin to your chest and slowly bend the elbows, letting the shoulders be the first to touch the floor. Come all the way down to your back. Remember to exit the pose the same way you entered it—mindfully and with the breath.

USTRASANA / CAMEL POSE

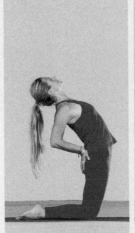

If you can't reach your heels, place a block on either side of the heels for the palms of the hands to rest.

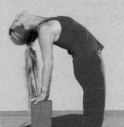

You can also do this pose with the toes tucked.

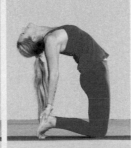

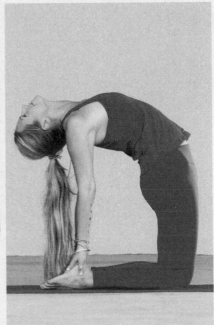

Come to your knees, double folding your mat or placing a blanket beneath the knees if your joints are sensitive. Keep the knees hip distance apart and line the hips up with the knees. Firm the inner thighs and keep pressing the hips forward as you lean back, reaching for your heels. You might have to bring the hips back just slightly to get there before you bring the hipbones forward again, lining them up with the knees. Let your head fall back and focus on creating space for the neck while softening the glutes. Stay for 5 slow breaths, or as long as you're comfortable.

SUPPORTED HEART OPENER

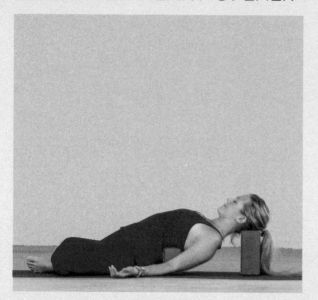 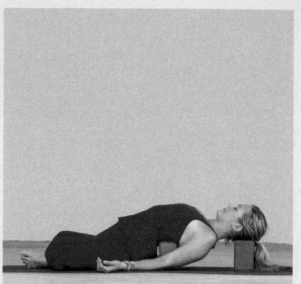

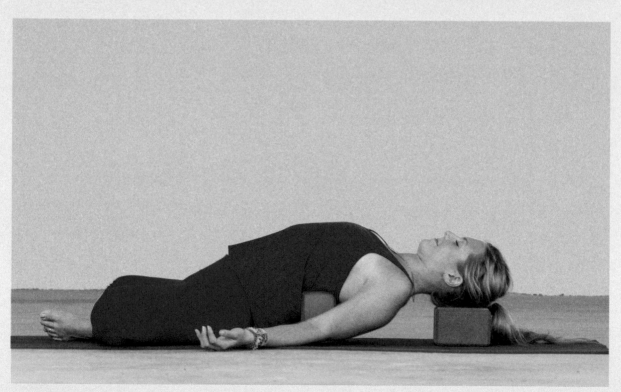

Come to a seated position with two blocks next to you. Place one of the blocks behind you on the mat on a medium level with the long end of the block lining up with the top of the mat. Place the other about the length of a block away, beginning on a high level. Lie down so that the edges of your shoulder blades drape over the first block and so that the second block ends up comfortably at the very back of your head. You can play around with the height of the block beneath your head until it's at a comfortable place (high, medium, or low). You can let your legs stay extended, or if you wish, connect the soles of the feet, allowing the knees to come out to the sides—whatever feels best to you. Let the arms rest down by your sides, palms facing up. Breathe deeply. Stay for a full minute or as long as you feel comfortable, rolling over to one side to come out of the pose when you're ready.

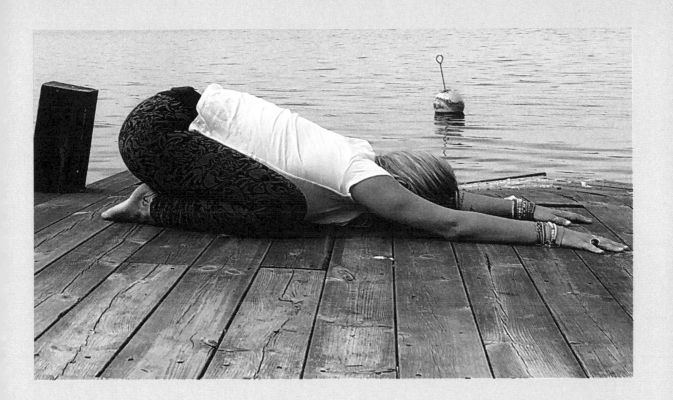

CHILD'S POSE / BALASANA

 Child's Pose is a beautiful place to slow down or take a little break between longer yoga sequences. Here you can allow the breath to slow down, and it's a safe place to ground yourself with the forehead touching the mat. Child's Pose is very healing for both the body and the soul, and is often used as a counterpose after advanced poses to rebalance before we continue to the next step. Come to Child's Pose as often as you like in a yoga class!

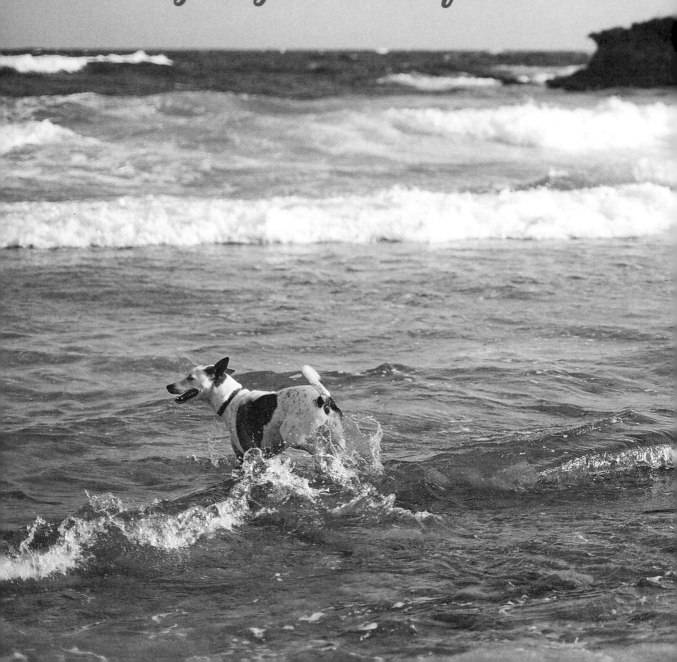

CHAPTER 5

Going with the flow

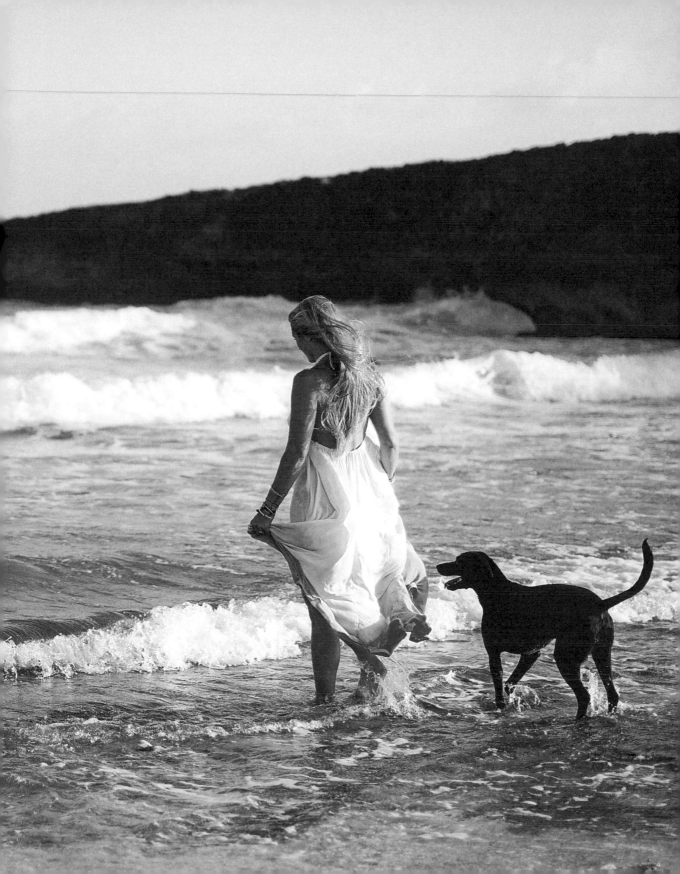

I practice yoga every single day, but my practice changes just like the seasons. During the peak of my most dynamic year thus far, when I was practicing like crazy and sweating and working so hard on the mat, I decided to start an Instagram account. I already had a Facebook page as a yoga teacher for my students to keep up with classes and changes, and I loved spreading inspiration and motivation for yoga online.

I was happy with my life in Aruba, classes were going well, and social media just seemed like a fun way to reach and connect with new people. I didn't have a plan for my Instagram account at all. I started posting little bits of my life—yoga on the beach, food that I ate, handstands, travels—and my following slowly grew. When I had two or three thousand followers, people started asking me for advice on yoga and yoga poses and I gladly replied.

A few months later Dennis and I hit a rough patch. This was a combination of different factors: He was very busy setting up his new skate shop, I was teaching a million classes a week, and we didn't have as much time together as we'd had before. At the same time some personal issues came up in my family, and instead of sharing that with Dennis and letting my problems bring us closer, I started to distance myself from him. What followed was the most challenging period of our relationship. We had never ever fought before, but all of a sudden we were fighting about little things all the time. I started spending more time going out with my girlfriends and acting a little bit crazy, and Dennis withdrew to his shop and stayed home with the dogs.

One day I was home, contemplating the difficult time we had found ourselves in, and to distract myself I reached for my phone to share a photo on Instagram of me doing a handstand. Normally I would caption the photos I shared with some information about the pose or just mention what a lovely day I was having. But at this very moment I wasn't having a lovely day. I was going through a shitty time. I don't know what came over me, but I started writing about my feelings—about the love and the pain and the struggles. And then I shared it with the world.

I didn't expect anything special, I just wanted to write down my thoughts, but instantly I started getting a big response. People commented on the post and told me they felt the same. I got e-mails from others sharing their own stories. What I had written resonated, and I realized: Many people out there are looking for inspiration, but the yoga pose is not what's important here. The love is important. Social media is

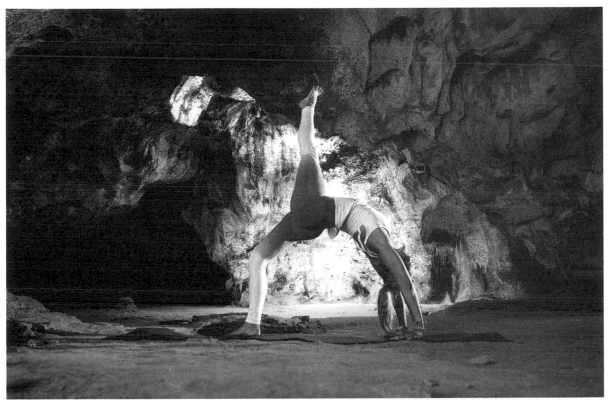

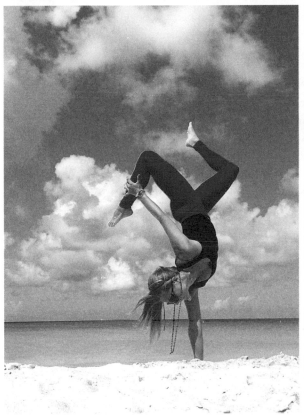

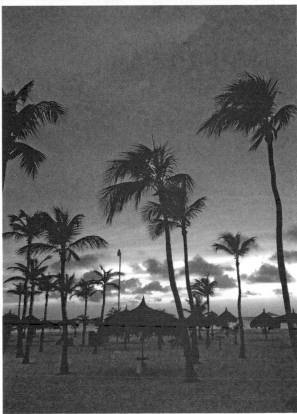

so full of negativity and unrealistic ideals that no one can live up to; people very rarely share what they actually feel.

I started posting more frequently, not caring very much about the photos I was sharing but focusing on my writing. If I had a bad day—working through trust issues in my relationship, for instance—I would sit down, meditate on it, and write my thoughts about trust down. Instead of keeping them to myself or in a journal, I shared them with the world. Through the pain I was in at the moment, a deep wisdom blossomed. Every day my following grew bigger and bigger, and not once did I stop to think about what I was creating or why. This was just an outlet for me to share my thoughts, bits of my day, and the wisdom I'd acquired throughout my life.

It was during this time that Dennis found yoga. He had never been particularly interested in yoga; he'd take my class once in a while, but it didn't really do anything for him. I think he still had the idea that yoga was something mainly for girls and for granola-eating hippies in hemp clothing (which it can be, and there is nothing wrong with that! But yoga is for everyone). One week Brock Cahill, someone I consider one of my biggest teachers for my physical practice, came to the island to lead a retreat with his wife. I'd never convinced Dennis to get into yoga before and I didn't expect that to change, but Dennis took his class and absolutely fell in love. Here was a guy who was stronger than Superman, did one-armed handstands, and seemed to effortlessly float above the ground—while keeping a smile on his face!

Dennis started taking my classes after that, and it turned out that the connection we thought we'd lost was still there, just waiting to be rekindled. Yoga brought us closer, and we worked through all the pain we'd experienced months earlier. It was around this time that my following on social media started to explode. I'd found my way back to that place of deep love and connection in my relationship, my practice was strong, classes were growing, and Dennis's shop was doing well; we had absolutely nothing to complain about. I could have gone back to my more shallow way of sharing with the world, but I didn't want to. I had no reservations at all about putting down my deepest thoughts, my ideas about life, and also my insecurities with the world.

My Instagram following blossomed into a community, and I continued sharing the happiness present in my yoga practice, our lives on the beach, food, but also real, human, raw emotion. I was amazed by the outpouring of love I was receiving and by how many people wanted to take my class. Over time I had started traveling to teach. The first class I ever taught internationally was in Orlando, Florida. We were going there for a Surf Expo, and some people had asked if I would consider teaching a class while I was there. I thought, *Sure, why not?* I had to google to find a studio that would take me in on such short notice, and then I shared the information on Instagram. I had maybe thirty or forty thousand followers at that time, and the workshop sold out right away. Actually, it ended up being the biggest workshop the studio had ever hosted! People were putting their mats down in the lobby and in the hallway leading into the studio because we had run out of space. The studio had no clue about who I was and were as surprised as I was to see people pouring in.

I was so nervous that my hands were shaking as I walked into the studio. It was one thing teaching my own students or tourists who came to visit the island or leading retreat groups, where I got to know people on a deeper level—no one really expected anything huge from me. But here was a big group of people that came from near and far specifically to see *me*. They had no idea if I was a good teacher or not. How could they? All they knew was that I was a person who liked to share inspirational things online. I felt that they expected me to be spectacular, something very special and out of the ordinary.

I sat down on my yoga mat and looked around. Fifty pairs of eyes looked back at me excitedly. I thought to myself: *I am who I am. I can only do my best.* So I did. I taught the best class I could possibly think of, and after two hours the class was deep in Savasana, many of them crying from the release of the practice. *I am good enough*, I thought. *I can do this.*

So I continued to travel, teach, and share my life with the world. Before I knew it, I had more than a million people following me every single day. This is when life started to get hectic. What once was a class of fifty people in a small yoga studio in Orlando turned into huge yoga events of five hundred to a thousand attendees. Suddenly life wasn't as calm and steady as I'd always wished it to be. I was so excited that people wanted me to come teach in different parts of the world that I started saying yes to everything. I went from teaching two to three retreat weeks a year to nine or ten. I taught workshops at events and festivals all over the United States, Canada, the Caribbean, Central America, Brazil, Scandinavia, and pretty much every single country in northern Europe. All of that in a year.

LOVING INSIGHTS

🕉 Let your practice evolve and change like the seasons.

🕉 Life gives us challenges to help us grow. Everything that comes our way is here for a reason. Don't shy away. Embrace the bad times as much as you do the good.

🕉 Value your relationships.

🕉 Be truthful. Tell the truth, tell the truth, tell the truth. To yourself. To your loved ones. To the world.

🕉 It does not matter what brings you to the mat. What matters is that you get there!

🕉 Nothing is more important than your own well-being. Sometimes saying no is caring for yourself.

🕉 Do your homework. What does your body need to heal?

🕉 Surrendering to what is and moving with life instead of against it is the key to happy living.

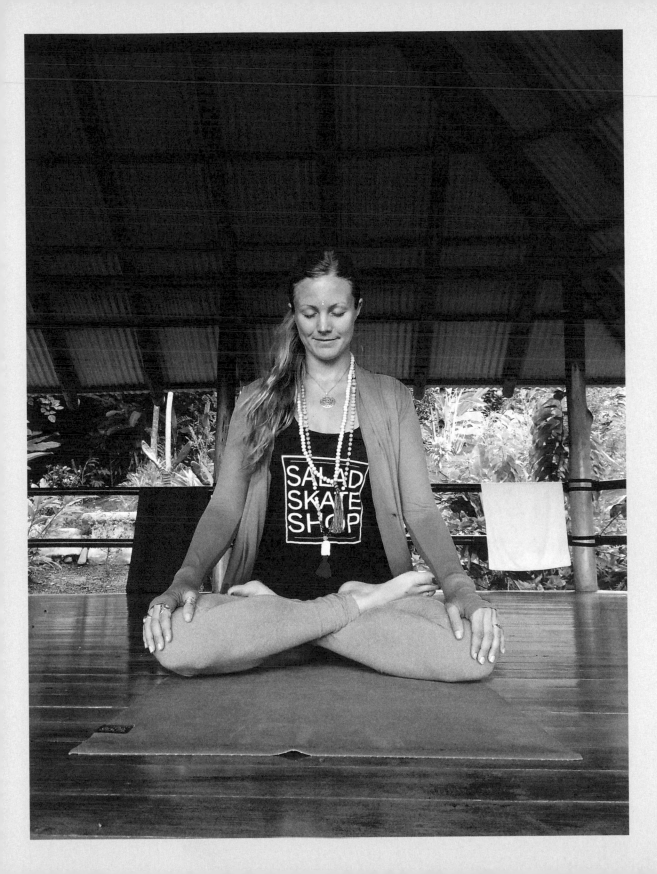

Traveling nonstop was a lot of fun in the beginning, and still is, but after a few months on the road I started to feel depleted. We were so busy traveling and teaching that I didn't have time for my own personal practice anymore. I'd do my best to sneak in some high-powered dynamic sequences when I had the time. I wanted to sweat and move as I always had, but there wasn't time for it anymore. I also did a lot of photo shoots at the time, which meant I'd put my body in difficult poses without warming up or preparing the way I normally would. All of this combined with something I'd been lucky enough to avoid for most of my life—stress—brought me back to the same place I had been years and years earlier: with back pain. We were on airplanes and in airports most of the time, sleeping in hotels, going from country to country, city to city, teaching every day.

One morning in San Francisco I awoke to the sound of my alarm clock, reached out to turn it off, and literally felt something snap in my neck. I had no idea what had happened. I couldn't move! I was in very little pain at first, but within minutes it was almost unbearable; I couldn't even get out of bed. And I had a jam-packed class that very afternoon! I knew at that moment that things were getting out of hand; I had become so caught up in teaching and trying to connect with everyone—I literally said yes to everyone who asked me to teach abroad—that my health and well-being had been compromised. This was not okay.

One of the most important rules that I live by is this: "To love others, you must first love yourself." You have to give yourself all the care you need! It's not just okay to be selfish, it's a necessity. If you run out of steam, how are you ever going to be of service to the world? If my body wasn't feeling good, how was I ever going to teach others to take care of theirs?

That day in San Francisco I made my way to the acupuncturist and was lucky enough to get a Thai massage from one of the most prominent therapists in the city. I felt better, but I walked into that class wearing thick knitted socks and a scarf (I was freezing!) and feeling so sad I could cry. I was teaching a handstand workshop and I couldn't even turn my head; someone had to help me sit down on my mat. The class went well anyway, I had friends demonstrate poses for me, and I built the class around what I personally needed the most at that moment: healing.

Sometimes life throws you both punches and curveballs, and you need to learn how to adapt to the flow of life.

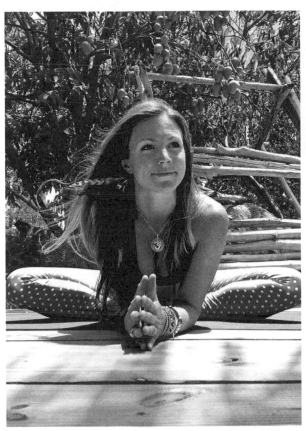
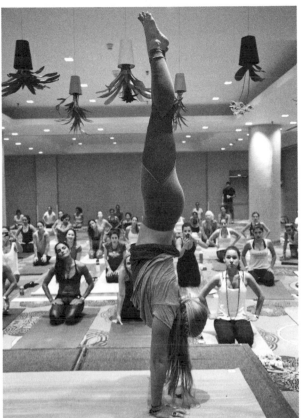
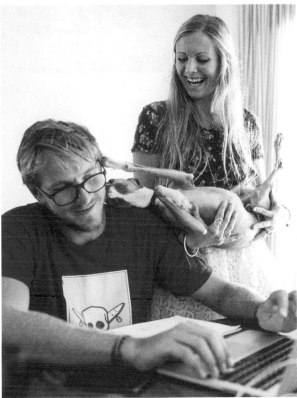
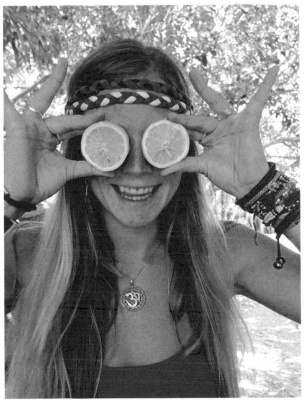

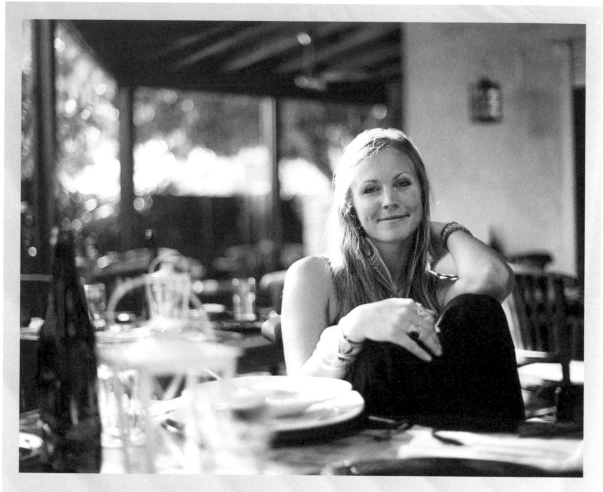

CARROT AND GINGER SOUP

2 pounds carrots, peeled and cut in rounds ❧ 3 large potatoes, peeled and sliced ❧ 1 big yellow onion, chopped ❧ 1 2-inch piece fresh gingerroot, peeled and chopped ❧ 4 cloves garlic ❧ 1 quart organic vegetable stock ❧ 1 (13.5-ounce) can organic coconut milk ❧ Salt and pepper to taste ❧ Cilantro for garnish

Place the carrots, potatoes, onion, ginger, and garlic in a large stockpot and cover with the vegetable stock. Bring to a boil and keep simmering on low heat until the vegetables and potatoes have softened. Add the coconut milk and bring to a boil again. Take the pot off the stove and use a hand blender or process in a blender a little at a time to mix well. Add salt and pepper to taste and garnish with cilantro.

_____

This soup is so nourishing! If you have a cold or if you're feeling a little low, add some more garlic and ginger and maybe a piece of chili pepper or two for an extra pick-me-up!

_____

From that day on, I changed my home practice from dynamic to restorative, and I made it a rule to get bodywork done—massage, acupuncture, energy work—once a week. We were all over the place and life was moving so fast around me; I had to adopt a practice that not only soothed my body but also my soul. I stopped thinking that my time on the mat had to look a certain way (aka flowy, advanced, and inverted) and focused on poses that would stretch my tight muscles in a safe way and would heal my back.

My homework will always be to heal my back; it's not a problem that suddenly will be fixed and go away. I need to keep my life stress free and my body healthy to feel good. That goes for all of us! This is why yoga is called a practice; we're never done.

Not a day goes by that I don't put my legs up against the wall (one of the most healing things you can do for a sensitive lower back). We all need to figure out what our yoga homework is; for some it's back pain, for others it's tight hamstrings, healing old injuries, a tense neck—what have you. Let your yoga heal you by adapting your practice to what you need during this moment of your life. I'm certain I will find my way back to a dynamic practice again (right now I'm someplace in between) because our yoga practice ebbs and flows like the tide. Surrendering to what is and moving with life instead of against it is the key. ❀

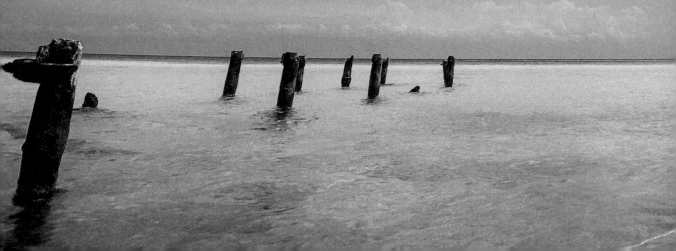

Restorative Yoga

Most of us lead busy lives. We rush from one place to another, taking in different impressions from our surroundings, constantly exposed to new people and situations. When was the last time you let yourself really relax?

Restorative yoga is a great complement to a vinyasa practice, as it gives us time and space to be present in the moment, let go of old tension, and heal our bodies from within. This chapter is about moving into safe, comfortable poses that you can stay in for a long time. Make sure that the temperature of the room you're in is comfortable (if you'd like, keep a blanket next to you to use for support or to cover yourself with if you get chilly), turn your phone off, and allow the breath to ground you in the here and now.

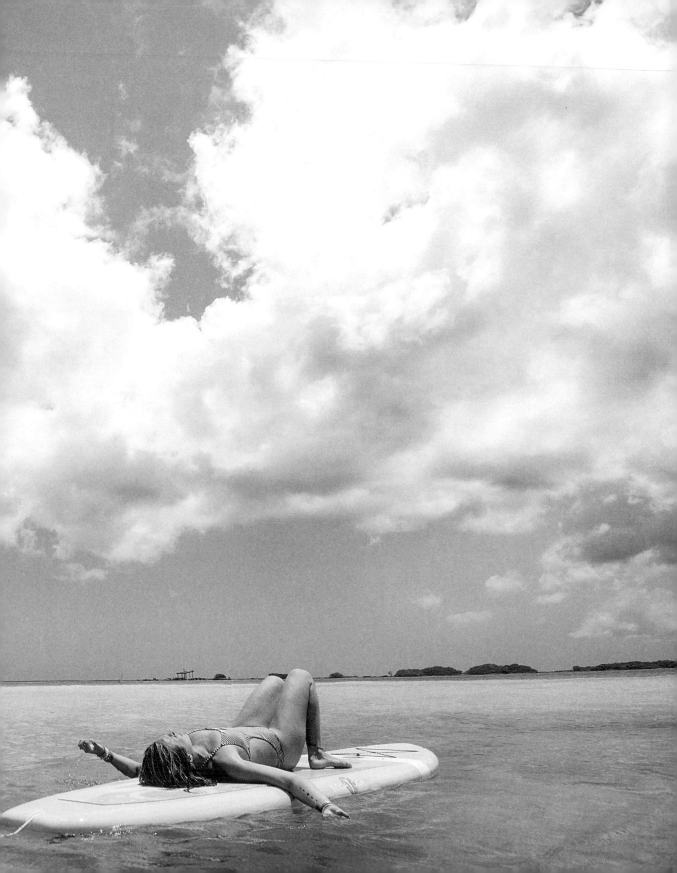

90-DEGREE LEGS

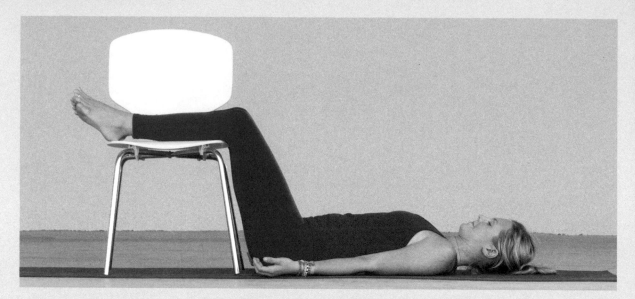

This is a very healing position for the entire spine, especially the lower back. If you're suffering from lower back pain, this is a great place to find release, but it's also excellent after a long day at the office. Place a chair on your yoga mat and lie down close to it. Bring your legs up to the seat of the chair. Bring your sit bones close enough to the chair that the shins become parallel to the floor. Let your calves rest comfortably on the chair and take the time you need to allow the lower back to fully relax. You can stay here for quite some time, breathing space into your lower back for as long as it feels good.

SEATED PIGEON ON A CHAIR

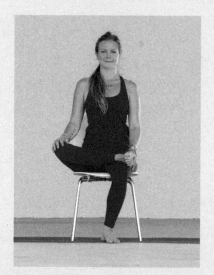

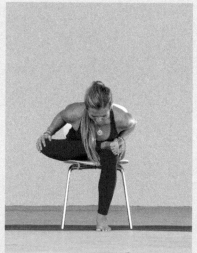

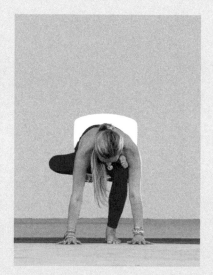

1 Sit on the edge of a chair, with your spine long. Place the right ankle on top of the left knee and flex the foot.

2 Gently bend over, folding forward. Relax the back of your neck and feel the soft stretch in the right hip and glute.

3 If you can, fold all the way down, placing your fingertips on the floor. Come back up with an inhale and switch legs when you're ready.

Here are a few general things to think about when you're practicing, regardless of the pose you're in:

꧁ Stay connected to the breath. When you feel your mind wandering, don't become frustrated but simply let that be a reminder for you to come back to the breath. Over and over again.

꧁ Keep the spine long. Think about the crown of your head as an extension of the spine—never tip the entire head back but be conscious to keep space for the neck.

꧁ Relax your face and your hands. When we're in long holds or deep stretches we sometimes unconsciously transfer tightness from one part of the body to another. Notice if you're making fists with your hands or clenching your jaw. Relax. Soften. Release.

꧁ Every time emotions pop up in our practice it means that your body is releasing emotional tension that's been stuck in certain body parts. It's absolutely natural to cry on your yoga mat—I do it all the time! Our yoga mat is a place of silence where we wholeheartedly can give ourselves the time we need to feel, and it's not uncommon for strong emotions to surface. Let it be! Cry when you need to. Allow the heart to open and your body to let go. Inhale to create space where space is needed. Exhale and release anything you might have been holding on to that is no longer of use. Keep breathing this way, and before you know it you've taken your yoga practice from the body all the way into your heart. In the heart, right here, is where true transformation happens.

VIPARITA KARANI / LEGS-UP-THE-WALL POSE

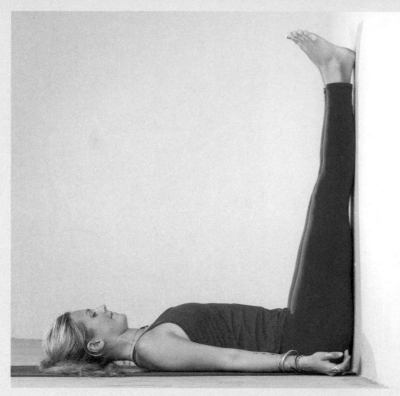

Come into a side squat with your outer hip facing the wall. Sit down and swing your legs up the wall and then wiggle your way as close as you can to the wall until your sit bones connect to it. If your hamstrings are very tight, you might want to keep your knees softly bent, or place a folded-up blanket beneath your lower back. Let your arms rest down by your sides, palms up. Breathe deeply.

OPEN LEGS

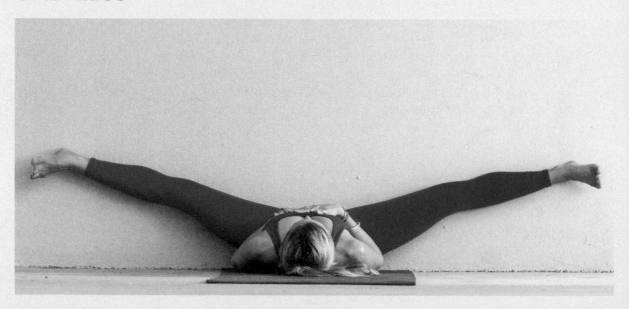

Open up your legs to the sides until you feel a good stretch in the inner thighs. Keep your toes active.

THE BUTTERFLY

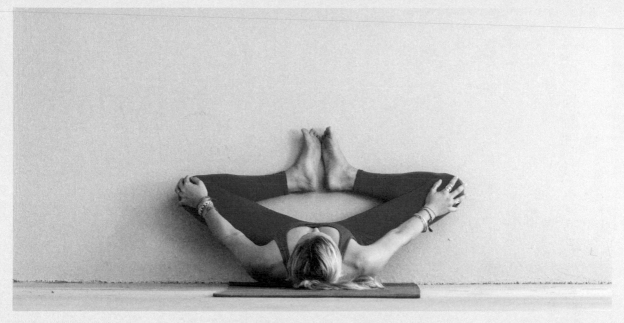

Bend your knees and bring the soles of your feet together. Allow your heels to draw closer toward your sit bones to deepen the stretch. If you like, gently press the palms of your hands toward the knees, bringing them slightly closer to the wall.

HIP OPENER

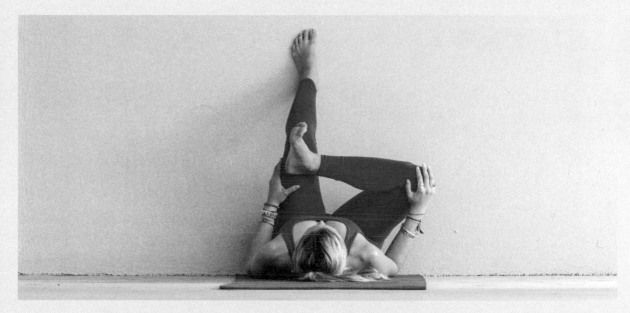

Come back to straight legs. Bend the right knee and place the right ankle directly above the left knee. Flex the foot. Gently bend the left knee, allowing the left heel to slide closer to the left sit bone. Pause where you feel a stretch in the right hip and glute. If you feel your tailbone lifting off the floor, soften the stretch, lengthen the tailbone down, and relax the lower back.

CHAPTER 6

Love over fear

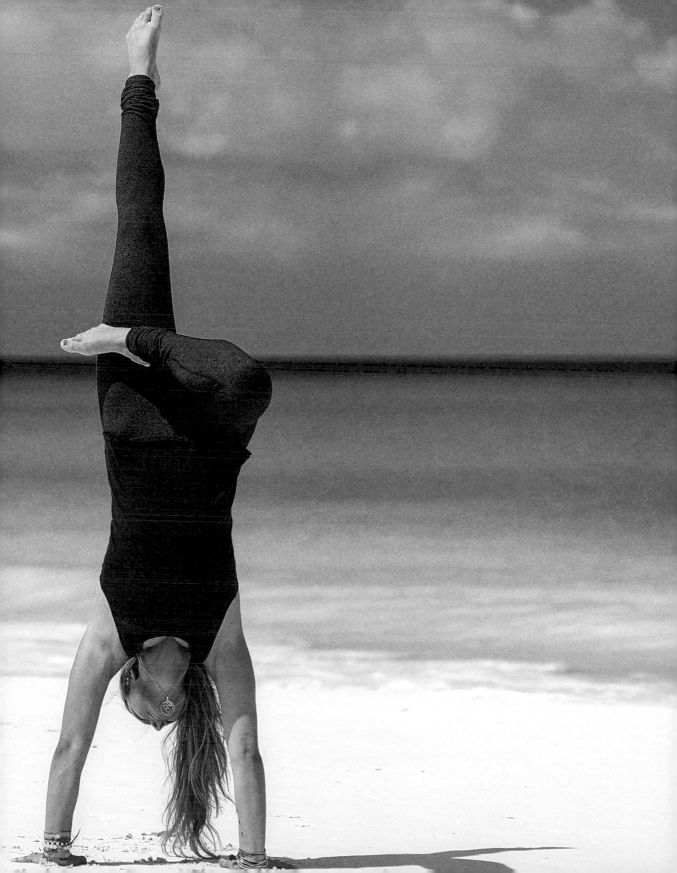

"I wanted to do something real, something substantial, something that was going to change the world—I just hadn't sat down to figure out exactly what it was yet."

Throughout these past years I've learned many lessons. I've learned how to carefully balance giving with receiving. I know now that I can't teach twenty-four classes a week and still stay sane. It's just not possible. I've learned to care for my body. I've learned to adapt my practice to the flow of life. I've learned I can't say yes to everything. Sometimes the best way to grow what you're doing and to stay aligned with your intentions is to say no! I've learned that miracles happen every day. You just have to keep your eyes open. I've learned how to embrace my past and how to take those lessons and turn them into wisdom. I've learned a lot, but most of all I've learned that to live a life that makes your heart sing, you need to let go of fear. We need to let go of fear—all of us, as a whole—and move the way love wants us to move.

I love to travel, but I can't do it nonstop. I've been moving around my entire adult life, hopping from country to country and changing direction with the wind. As things started to speed up, I knew I had to align my intentions with what it was I wanted to create. This is how life works: When you're on a roll, you're on a roll. If you believe and expect things to come your way, they will, and sometimes we manifest things more quickly than we could ever have imagined. That's why it's so important to sit down and decide what it is we want to manifest in our lives before things start moving so quickly we no longer control the steps that we take. I found myself with all these blessings in life: a beautiful partner; a career that allows me to share my passion for yoga and happy living with the world; and of course, a community of people who are on this path with me! I knew the following I had created was special; my main intention was always to stay real and true to who I am, and to help people find the same love for themselves at their core. It's all about love. Forgiveness. Being kind. I wanted to do something real, something substantial, something that was going to change the world—I just hadn't sat down to figure out exactly what it was yet. From trial and error I knew that in order to make this happen I had to let go of my deepest fears.

Since I started to embrace this path, I've had to overcome some serious fears of mine. First, I am scared shitless of public speaking. You might not be able to imagine that, since I teach yoga for a living (teaching is pretty much speaking to the public), but it took me a long time to get comfortable speaking in front of a group. I used to be so nervous I was nauseated before every class. On a bad day I'd go over in my head all the possible things that could go wrong: *What if I forget the words? What if I fall over?*

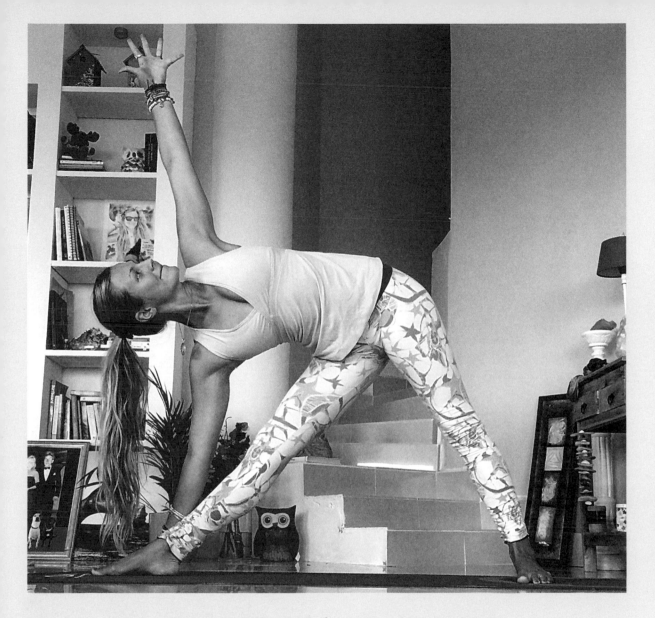

There are many different kinds of yoga mats to choose from. Pick one that fits your lifestyle! I travel a lot, so I have a super-thin, lightweight foldable mat that I take everywhere I go and a thick, heavy yoga mat at home that always stays put. If you have sensitive knees I recommend a thicker mat so you have good support for your joints (and keep a blanket by your side!). Most important, the mat should be a good size for you and you shouldn't slip when you practice. If you're tall, you might need an extra-long mat, and if you have broad shoulders, you might need a wider mat. It's better to spend a little extra on a good quality mat than to buy a cheap mat that'll leave you sliding all over the moment you start to sweat (one of the most common poses, Downward-Facing Dog, is super tricky if your hands are sliding!). These days you can also find a great selection of organic and recycled mats. A quality mat will last you a long time, so a good yoga mat is a great investment!

121

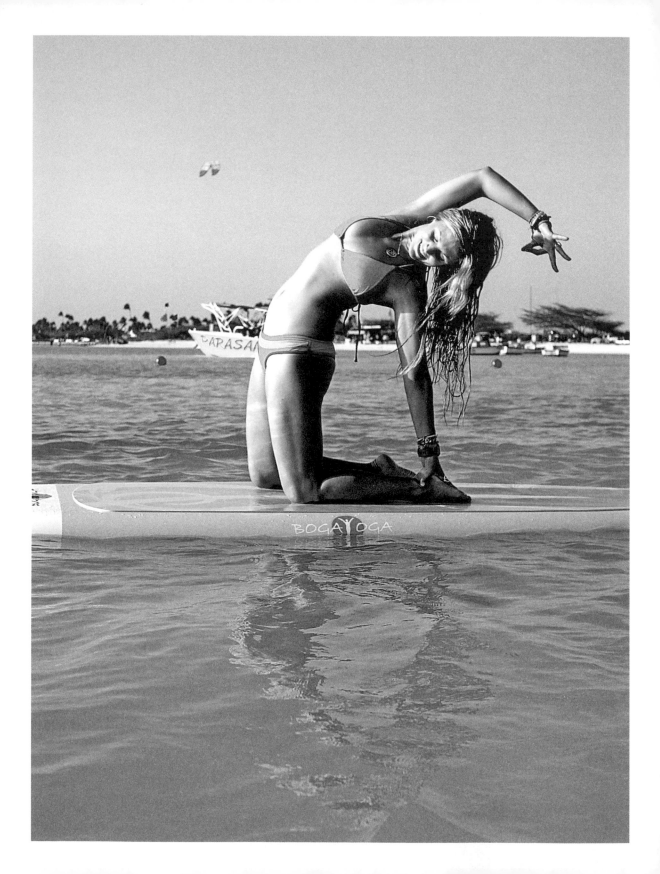

"I would always come back to the same thought:
Do your best."

What if someone asks me a question I can't answer? What if they all laugh at me because I'm so terrible? I would always come back to the same thought: *Do your best.* Who is judging me here, really? No one judges us harder than we do ourselves. The expectations and judgments I was feeling all came from me. In the end I would think: *Keep going forward. Don't go back.* Then I would step into the class and simply do what I had to do, because if I decided then and there not to teach the one class that scared me the most, I wouldn't have learned all the things I needed to learn. I look back at my first year of teaching and can see the importance of those difficult classes. Every time I pushed through the fear of failure and taught the class, I took one step up the ladder that has taken me to where I am today. We need to keep moving up, up, up. The funny thing is, no one ever even knew I was nervous! That's the thing about teaching yoga; people aren't really there for you. They're there for themselves. All of us have our own path and our own issues; most of us spend so much time worrying about ourselves that we rarely notice what's going on with other people. This is how I finally overcame my fear of teaching; I knew that if I focused on my nerves, I would never truly see the people in front of me. If I gave those people 100 percent of my attention, as a good teacher always should, I wouldn't be able to worry about how my voice sounded or if my sequencing was good enough. I started to relax and my true voice as a teacher came out. My teaching improved dramatically. There is no difference between Rachel Brathen the person and Rachel Brathen the teacher—it's all me. And this shows in my teaching.

There is a twist to all of this, of course. For every fear you move past, there is a bigger one lurking around the corner. I went from being nervous about teaching small, local classes on the island where I lived to being nervous about teaching big classes across the globe. As a new teacher in Aruba, I watched the size of my classes grow, and even though I got more and more confident, my stomach would still churn if I walked into the studio and there were twenty-five people instead of the anticipated ten. After a while I was teaching so many classes in a week it became my new normal to move through a new fear every day. Classes grew and I overcame my fear of teaching big groups. Well-known teachers came to the island, which made me nervous, of course. *What if I'm not good enough to teach a teacher?* I came back to that simple philosophy of mine, did my absolute best, and overcame that fear, too. We are all teachers and students, and whatever judgment we put on others is usually directed at ourselves.

LOVING INSIGHTS

🕉 Balance giving with receiving.

🕉 Miracles happen every day!

🕉 Move past your fears. If it scares you, do it!

🕉 Feeling nervous is a sign that what you're doing is important. Feeling nervous means you're breaking new ground. Use it to your advantage!

🕉 Find your voice. Whatever you're doing, let the real you shine through. Instead of imitating others, figure out what makes you unique and let that be at the core of your work.

🕉 When opportunity comes knocking, open the door! Trust in your own ability to create magic.

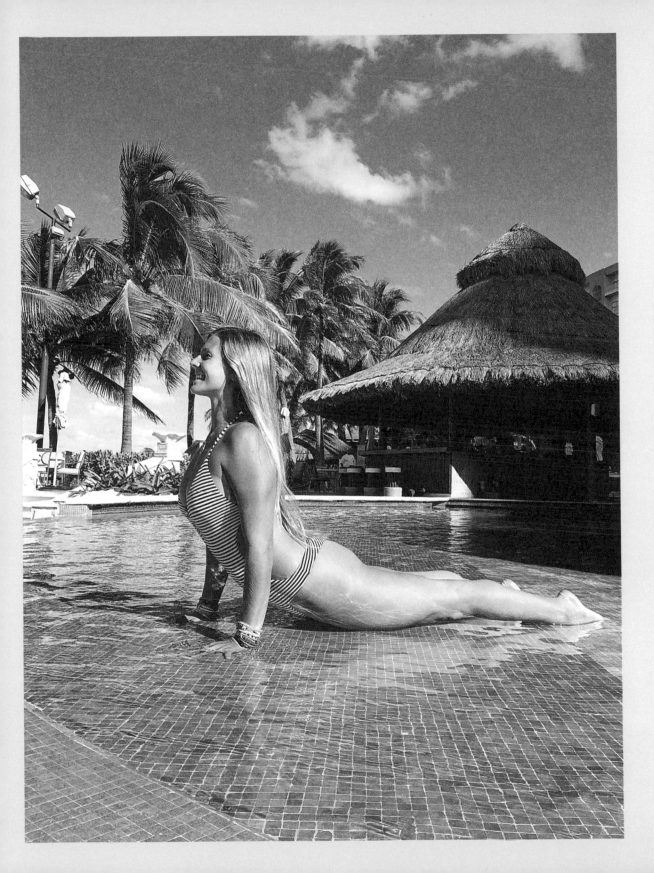

*"If doing something new doesn't scare you
at least a little, it's not worth doing."*

I have had to overcome many, many fears along the way; for every big new thing there has been this little voice in my head saying, *This is scary*. We all have this inner cautionary voice, and succeeding and evolving is all about how well we manage it. I started teaching at big events involving more than five hundred people at a time—that was scary. I started sharing my classes online—that was scary. I taught at the biggest yoga festival in the world—that was scary. I shot a DVD—that was scary. Reporters for big magazines interviewed me—that was scary. I flew across the world for meetings with powerful executives about my brand—that was scary. I was interviewed on TV—that was scary. I demonstrated yoga on stage with the king and queen of Holland on live TV in front of ten thousand people. *That* was scary! I moved to a tiny island just to be with a man I'd known for only five days. I said yes when that same man, who turned out to be the love of my life, asked me to marry him. I signed the contract for our very first house. I started a business. I wrote a book. All of these things have been the scariest and most wonderful moments of my entire life. I said good-bye to people in my life that I never in a million years thought I'd have to say good-bye to. I found myself faced with a thousand scary moments that in the big scheme of things make up our lives, and I chose love. I chose love. That is all.

And here is one of the scariest things of all: welcoming all of the beautiful souls who have made a decision to come take my classes throughout the years. Beautiful, beautiful souls, all showing up with open hearts, just to listen to what I have to say. Just to connect. To practice. To move. To hug. Brave, strong souls who have allowed themselves to be vulnerable, who have written me, called me, or visited from afar just to say hello. Intimacy and vulnerability are both scary things to show to the world. Here's the thing, though; if doing something new doesn't scare you at least a little, it's not worth doing. The marvelous moments, the situations we find ourselves in that make us grow and evolve and expand our hearts—all are going to be covered with a thin veil of fear. We are stepping into the unknown, and this means different things to all of us. Moving with love instead of fear takes courage, but on the other side of it lies liberation. Enlightenment. Joy. Happiness. Healing. Acceptance. Surrender. Gratitude. Magic. Freedom.

A perfect place to practice letting go of fear is on the yoga mat. What poses scare you? For many it's arm balances, advanced poses, and inverted poses, poses that involve your going upside down. Inversions can be terrifying; they are a giant step into the unknown when we first start practicing them and literally turn life as we know it upside down. But

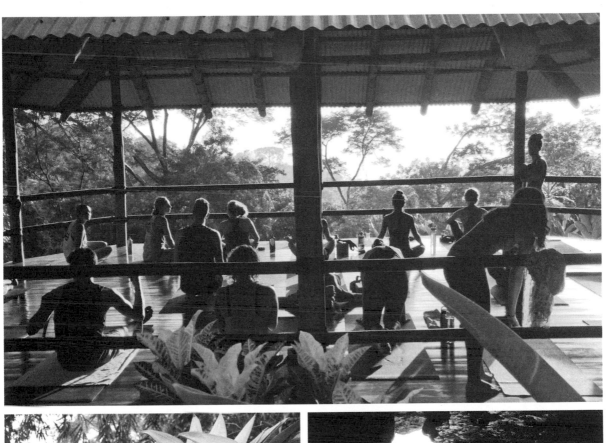

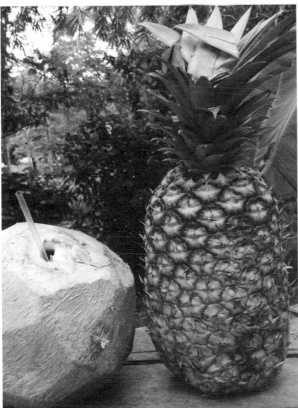

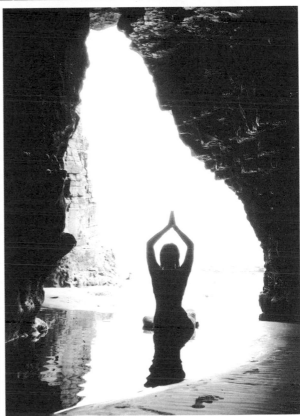

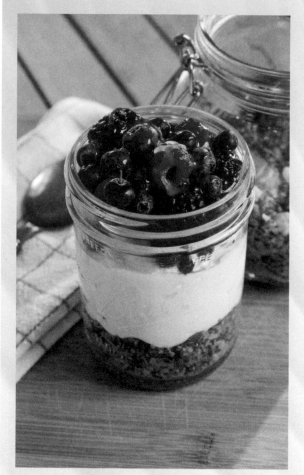

UPSIDE-DOWN GRANOLA IN A JAR

GRANOLA
2 tablespoons coconut oil ✿ 1 tablespoon maple syrup ✿ 1 cup oats ✿ ½ cup shredded coconut ✿ ½ cup chopped hazelnuts ✿ ½ cup slivered almonds ✿ ½ cup chopped dried figs ✿ ½ cup chopped dried apricots ✿ ½ teaspoon chia seeds ✿ Pinch Himalayan salt ✿ Pinch cinnamon

TOPPING
Yogurt (Greek, Turkish, or vegan coconut yogurt!) ✿ Blueberries ✿ Raspberries ✿ Blackberries ✿ Raw honey

Start by making the granola. Preheat the oven to 350°F. In a small bowl, mix the coconut oil and the maple syrup and set aside. In a large bowl, mix all the dry ingredients together with the dried fruits and then add the coconut/maple syrup mix. Mix well—use your hands if you like! Put the mixture in an oven-safe pan and bake until your entire kitchen smells delicious (or until the mixture has turned golden). Let it cool.

Put the granola at the bottom of a mason jar, fill the jar with yogurt, and add a mix of berries. Drizzle honey on top and enjoy heaven in a jar!

You can put pretty much anything in your granola; different kinds of seeds, nuts, and dried fruits. Or why not add pieces of dark chocolate after the mixture has cooled?

CHOCOLATE SHAKE, YOGA-GIRL STYLE!

1 banana ✿ 3 tablespoons almond butter ✿ 2 pitted dates ✿ 2 tablespoons raw cacao powder ✿ Handful of Brazil nuts ✿ 1 teaspoon hempseed ✿ Almond milk ✿ Few sprigs of mint

This smoothie is a great afternoon boost! Place all the ingredients in a high-speed blender and add just enough almond milk to get the blender going and enough ice to make sure the texture resembles a chocolate milk shake. Garnish with hempseed and mint leaves.

"You have to do the work. No one is going to do it for you. Don't hold back."

these poses are so empowering; they create a deep sense of accomplishment and confidence. The strength I have on the mat and the space I've created in my body are the result of a lot of hard work, but mostly . . . a lot of letting go. We hold so much emotion in the body. Practicing yoga is releasing—that's why it's so difficult! Not because we move in different ways or inhale to lift this and exhale to lower that. It's scratching at the surface of what you don't want to see; it's revealing all the fears and judgments you have buried deep inside yourself. It's connecting to what's really true. And yes, along the way we might pick up some strength and flexibility and handstands and backbends and arm balances—all a bonus. But this is not the purpose of our practice, the reason we keep returning to the mat every damn day. As I move deeper and deeper into my own inversion practice, I move deeper and deeper into self-love. As I build the strength to balance steadily on my hands, I build the strength to face whatever the world throws at me. As I release tension from the hips, shoulders, and hamstrings, I release fear, frustration, sadness. Little by little I release the need to control. As I learn to surrender on the mat, I learn to surrender to the present moment. This is the practice. It's accessible to you, to everyone, right here, right now—but you have to do the work. No one is going to do it for you. Don't hold back.

There are still things that scare me, of course, but I've made it a rule: Whenever I feel that flutter of fear at the pit of my stomach, I *have* to do it. If the thought of it makes me nervous, I have to say yes. This is how I continue to grow as a teacher, as a student, and as a human being. The idea of writing a book used to feel daunting, but just look at me now. I get approached regularly about lectures, and up until very recently this was something that made my palms sweat just from thinking about it. *Public speaking? Me? Never!* The thing about life is, you get what you need. Not what you want. And everything happens at the right time. As I finished writing this chapter, I got a call from an inspirational event management company asking me to lecture in front of an audience of seven hundred people about the book and my life as a traveling yoga instructor. I immediately said no—no way. I teach yoga, I don't lecture, I said. It's just not for me. I hung up the phone feeling a bit queasy from the mere idea, and turned back to my computer. The first thing my eye caught was the title of this very chapter: Love over fear. Love. Over. Fear. I'd just written an entire chapter about moving past your fears, and here I was, turning down opportunities because I was scared? I knew what I had to do. I called the company back and accepted. I said yes. I chose love. ✺

Inversions and Handstands

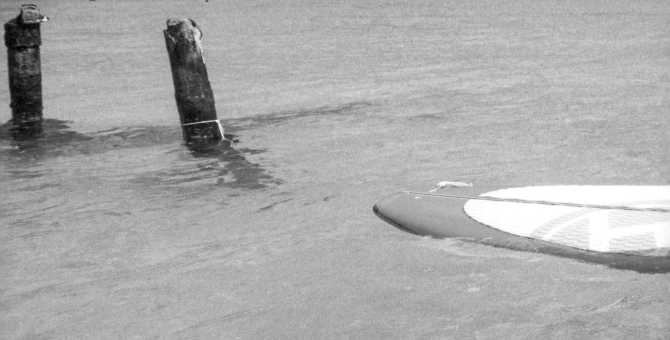

Yoga is never ending—that's why it's called a practice. When you feel ready to take your physical practice to the next level, you can start to move toward more advanced poses such as arm balances and inversions—if you feel drawn to them!

Advanced poses that require us to stay upside down or balance on our hands are not the purpose of our yoga practice, although these types of poses are becoming increasingly popular. Handstands and other inversions help you to build strength and balance, but it's important to remember that the poses themselves are not the reason we step on the mat over and over again. We are here to cultivate peace. Focus. Calm.

Advanced poses can help you get there (finding peace while inverted is deeply rewarding), but make sure you don't become frustrated when these poses don't happen for you right away. Continue taking deep breaths and know that we all begin from where we are. These are difficult poses, and while they may come easily for some, most people need years of practice to become comfortable in them. Try to enjoy the journey without becoming too attached to the result!

Learning how to handstand was a big moment for me. It wasn't just exciting and challenging, but it also helped me build a lot of core strength, which in turn supported my troublesome lower back. Handstands also gave me great confidence and a feeling of *I can!* The key to finding balance upside down lies in trusting in your own ability and believing in yourself. Find your center. Choose love over fear and give it a try!

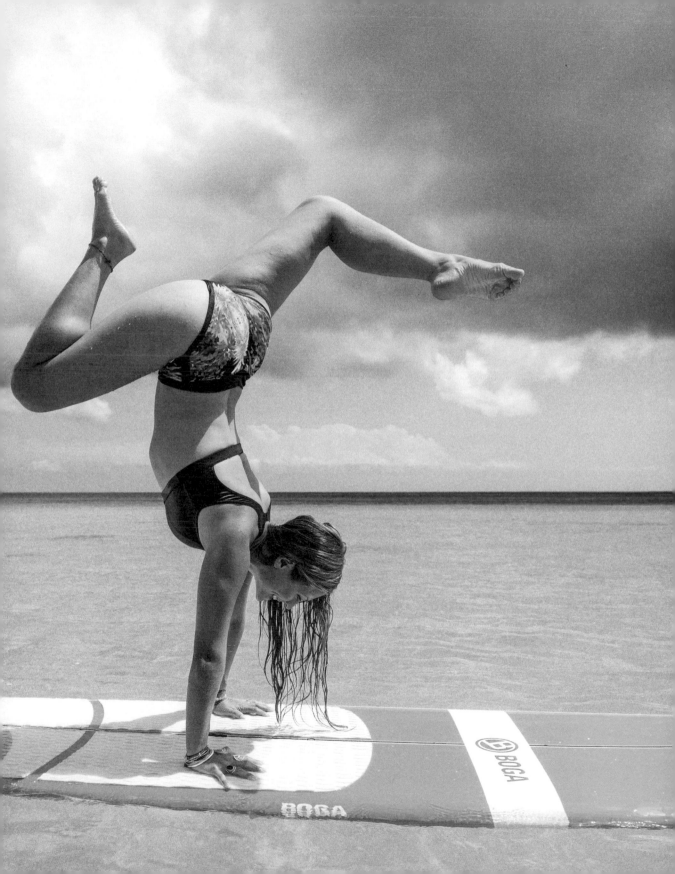

SALAMBA SIRSASANA / SUPPORTED HEADSTAND

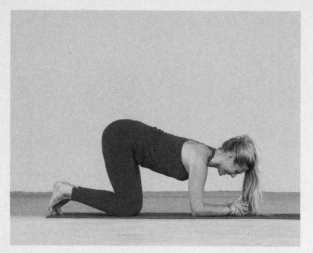

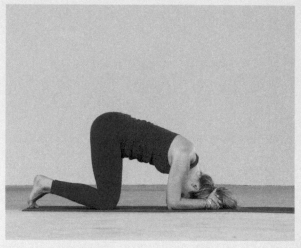

1 If you are new to headstands, practice them against the wall! Come to your knees on the mat. Begin by checking the space between your elbows so that they line up with your shoulders (you want to be able to wrap your fingers around the edges of your elbows). A common mistake is moving the elbows out to the sides, creating a space that's too wide in between. If you do this, you lose the frame of the upper body that supports you in this headstand! Measure the proper space, then keep the elbows where they are.

2 Interlace the fingers and tuck the last pinkie finger in so you have a steady base. Press the forearms down and then place the very center of the crown of the head down, letting the hands just barely connect to the back of your head for support.

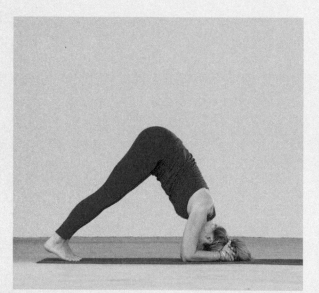

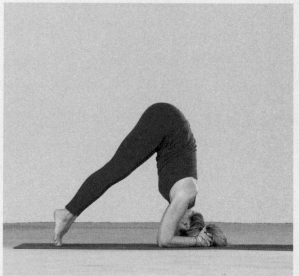

3 Tuck your toes under and lift your knees off the floor. This is step one of our preparation for headstand, so if you're just beginning to learn this pose I suggest you stay here. Press the forearms to the mat, draw the shoulders off the neck, and broaden the upper back. Start to slowly walk your feet in toward your elbows.

4 Try keeping as little pressure on the crown of your head as possible. Use the strength of the shoulders and the core here; don't collapse your weight on the crown of your head! Keep the neck long and walk your feet as close in toward the elbows as you can, until your hips stack on top of your shoulders. Now you're halfway to headstand! There is no kicking or flinging the legs involved here, but keep shifting your weight forward until you feel the feet getting lighter.

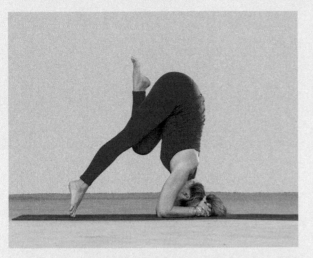

5 Now, lift one foot off the floor, pulling the knee in toward the chest. Bring the foot back down, and try the other side. Work on shifting from left to right, and with a little bit of practice you'll soon find the balance to lift both feet off the mat.

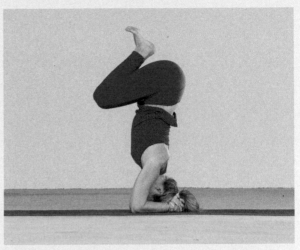

6 Keep the knees in toward your chest for a while, connecting to the breath.

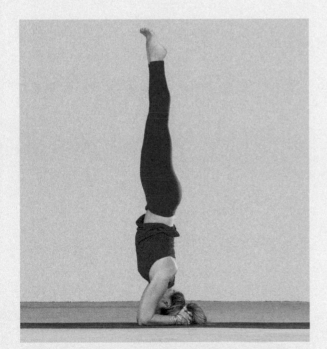

7 When you're ready, start extending both legs straight up toward the sky. Ground down through the forearms, draw the ribs inward, engage the inner thighs, and work on sending energy all the way to the tips of the toes. Lengthen the tailbone toward the heels, activate your core, and breathe deeply.

If you're unsure of where the exact center point of the crown of your head is, place the base of your palm in between the eyebrows. Where the middle finger reaches the top of the head is usually the very center! You can also try balancing a block or a book on the top of your head while keeping your spine long. The place where the block stays in balance without falling is your center point. Make sure you find the correct placement of the head in headstand to avoid unnecessary compression of the neck.

8 Make your way down the same way you came up, one step at a time. Rest in Child's Pose (see page 99) with the arms stretched out in front of you for as many breaths as you spent upside down.

PINCHA MAYURASANA / FOREARM STAND

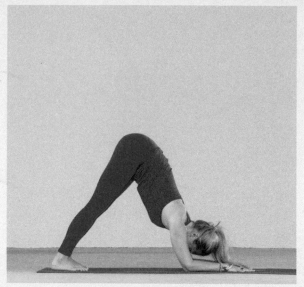

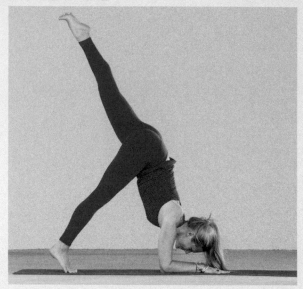

1 Begin in Dolphin Pose. This is just like Downward-Facing Dog, but with the forearms on the floor. Measure the space between the elbows the same way you did for the supported headstand. Draw the shoulder blades down, keep the neck long, and start to walk the feet in toward the elbows.

2 When you feel like you can't walk the feet any closer, lift one leg off the floor. Keep the hips squared and gaze slightly forward.

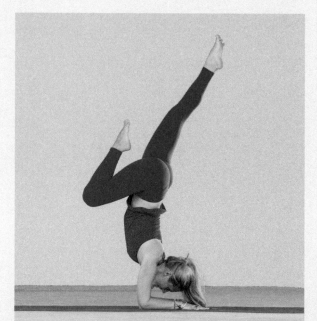

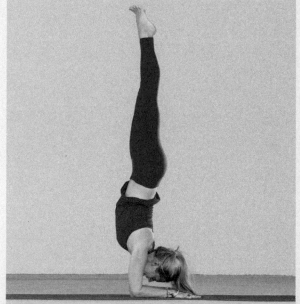

3 Come to the ball of the standing foot, bend the knee, and kick up gently. If you're a beginner, do this at the wall! Only kick as high as you can without there being any fear of falling involved, so go easy and stay patient. Once you get the hips above the shoulders, pull the lower knee in toward the chest and use the leg as leverage to find your balance. Use your fingertips as brakes!

4 When you've found your balance and feel steady, bring both legs straight up toward the sky. Connect the two big toes, engage the inner thighs, and draw the lower ribs in to connect to the transverse abdominals. Keep creating space for the neck and send energy to the tips of the toes. When you're ready, come down and rest in Child's Pose (page 99).

EKA PADA GALAVASANA / FLYING PIGEON POSE

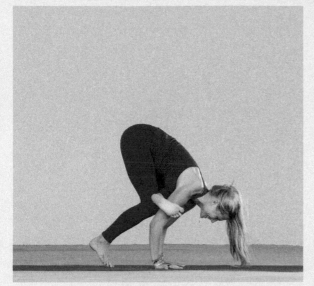

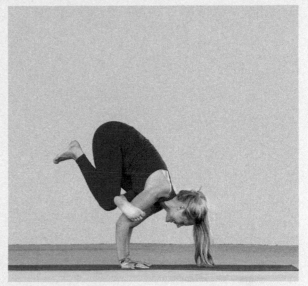

1 Come to a standing position. Balancing on the right foot, place the left ankle directly above the right knee. Flex the left foot and fold forward, placing the hands on the mat shoulder distance apart. You want the shinbone to press against the back of the right arm, as high as it goes, and then use the left foot to wrap around the right triceps. Press the tops of the toes to the back of the arm so you feel almost as if the foot is glued to the arm; this is what will keep you steady when you take off! Lift the hips high and start shifting some weight into the tips of the fingers.

2 Let your heart guide you forward until you feel the right foot becoming lighter and lighter. With time and practice you'll be able to fly!

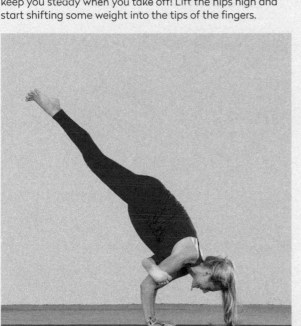

When it comes to hand balances and inversions, be patient and focus on one step at a time. The first step to mastering an advanced position is deciding to give it a try, but don't rush the process. Focus on the path, not the destination! Advanced poses are fun and challenging, but they are not the purpose of our practice. Focus on your breath and pause wherever it feels right to you. Most arm balances and inversions require lots of time and practice, so listen to your body, go easy, and remember to come right back up with a smile every time you fall.

3 Keeping both hips squared, engage the back of the right leg and start to extend it straight up and back behind you. Rotate the inner thigh toward the sky, press the thumbs to the floor, and keep a steady gaze.

ADHO MUKHA VRKSASANA / HANDSTAND

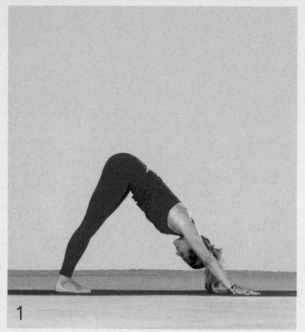

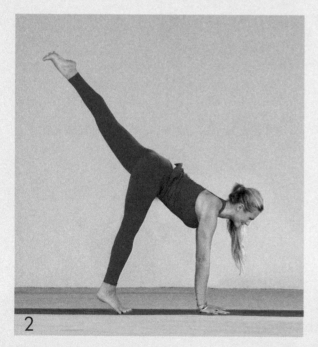

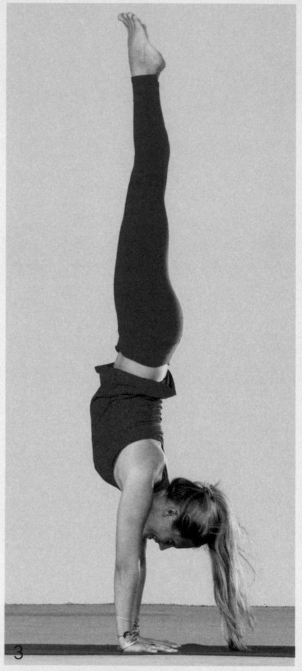

Begin in Downward-Facing Dog. Take a step forward and lift one leg up. You want the shoulders to align with the wrists and the thumbs pressing down on the mat. Wrap the triceps back, keep the hips squared, and engage the lifted leg. Gaze forward and come to the ball of the standing foot. Bend the bottom knee and kick up off the floor, bringing the heel toward the sit bone. Try this a couple of times, soft kicks off the floor without too much expectation of what your handstand kicks should look like. In the beginning, focus on simply lifting the leg off the floor! If you're worried about falling over, use a wall. Once you find your balance with the hips stacked over the shoulders, extend both legs straight up toward the sky. Pull the lower belly in; you want to feel your core engaged! Think about decreasing the space between the floating ribs and the two frontal points of the hips. Actively press the floor away from you and breathe!

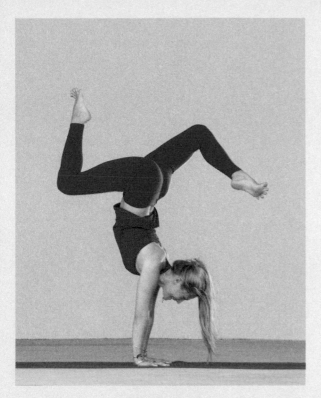

IMPORTANT THINGS TO THINK ABOUT WHEN WORKING ON YOUR HANDSTAND:
- Shoulders line up with wrists
- Spread the fingers wide
- Press the thumbs and the index fingers down properly
- Arms are straight, but don't lock the elbows in!
- Squared hips
- Top leg straight and strong—don't bend the knee of the lifted leg
- Shoulders away from the ears
- Gaze forward so you know where you're going!
- Kick yourself in the butt (heel to sit bone) to make balancing easier

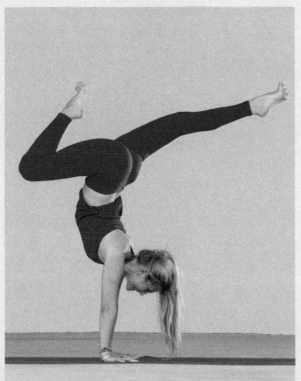

If you've been practicing your handstands for a while and feel comfortable balancing upside down, you can start working on different variations. Try bending your knees into your chest, or split your legs open! Breathe deeply and smile.

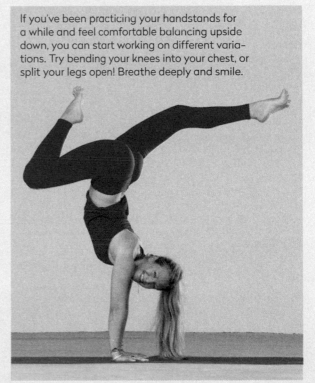

ADHO MUKHA VRKSASANA / HANDSTAND AGAINST THE WALL

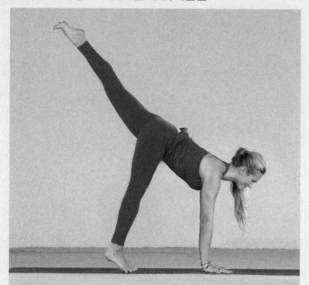

1 Begin in Downward-Facing Dog facing the wall. Take a big step forward and lift one leg, the same way as shown on page 136.

Engage your core. Keep the pelvis neutral. Try not to arch the back.

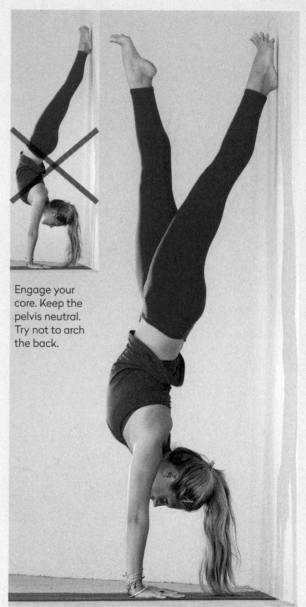

Try to get away from the wall by using these tips. When you start kicking up to handstand, be very patient and listen to your body. You will most likely not kick very high in the beginning as you want to avoid falling over or flipping into Wheel Pose (this is a conscious transition, not an appropriate way to fall out!). When we fall over, we twist from the center of the body, cartwheeling out of the pose to land on our feet. With time and practice, you will be able to kick up higher with more control. When your hips start aligning above the shoulders, you'll experience your first moments of balancing upside down. Learning handstand requires working on both alignment and technique, as well as building strength. It can be quite a long process, so make sure you enjoy yourself and have fun along the way!

2 Kick up and bring the legs to the wall, but once you have your balance, allow only one heel to rest against it for support. Keep the other heel in line with the knee and the knee lining up with the hips. Pull the lower ribs in and lengthen the tailbone toward the sky so that you teach your body the proper alignment of the handstand even though you're using the wall for support. Try bouncing the supported heel away from the wall for a second or two, playing around with your balance. Switch heels and try again! Never let both heels rest against the wall; this will make you collapse from the ribs, creating a big dip in the lower back. Use the wall for support in the beginning, but don't rely on it! Get to the middle of the room as soon as you feel more stable.

BAKASANA / CROW POSE

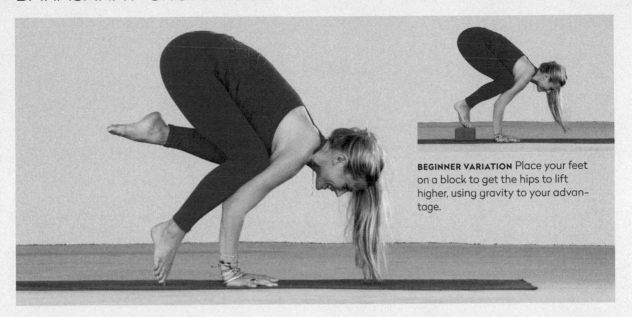

BEGINNER VARIATION Place your feet on a block to get the hips to lift higher, using gravity to your advantage.

1 Come into a squatting position. Place the palms of the hands shoulder distance on the floor, lift the hips up high, and bring the knees as high up the back of the arms as you can, toward the armpits. Round the upper back slightly, gaze forward, and let the heart follow the gaze.

Looking forward will help keep you from falling over! Keep the toes on the mat and start shifting more and more weight forward. When the toes start feeling light, bring one heel in toward the sit bone.

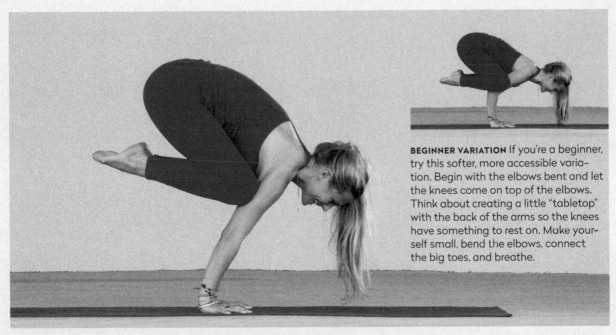

BEGINNER VARIATION If you're a beginner, try this softer, more accessible variation. Begin with the elbows bent and let the knees come on top of the elbows. Think about creating a little "tabletop" with the back of the arms so the knees have something to rest on. Make yourself small, bend the elbows, connect the big toes, and breathe.

2 When you feel ready for takeoff, lift both feet off the floor and bring the heels in toward the sit bones. Keep the two big toes together, engage your core, and relax the neck. Work your way toward straight arms (also called Crane Pose) if you like, using your core strength to hug in and lift up, pressing down through the palms of the hands to straighten the arms slowly.

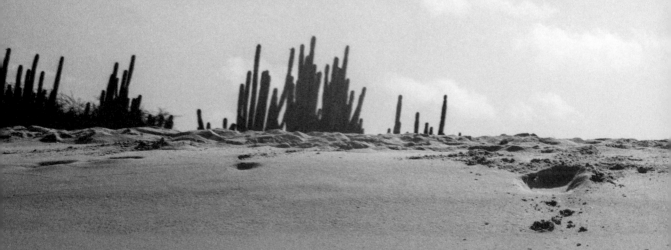

CHAPTER 7

Moments of silence

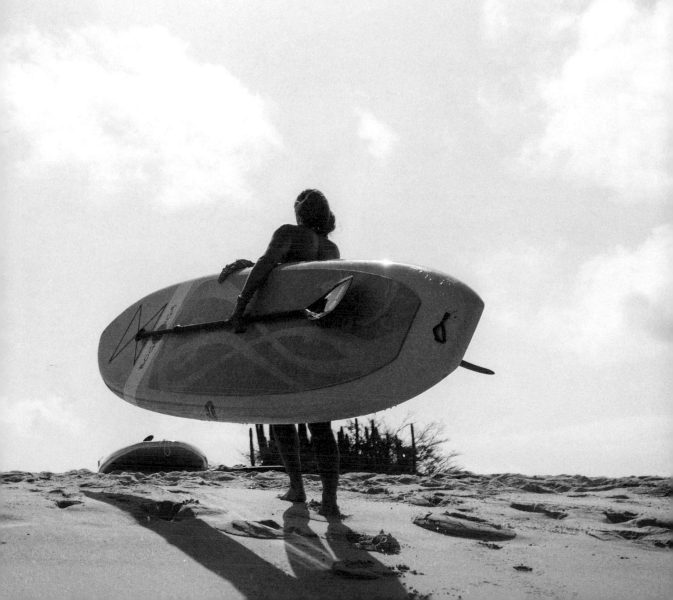

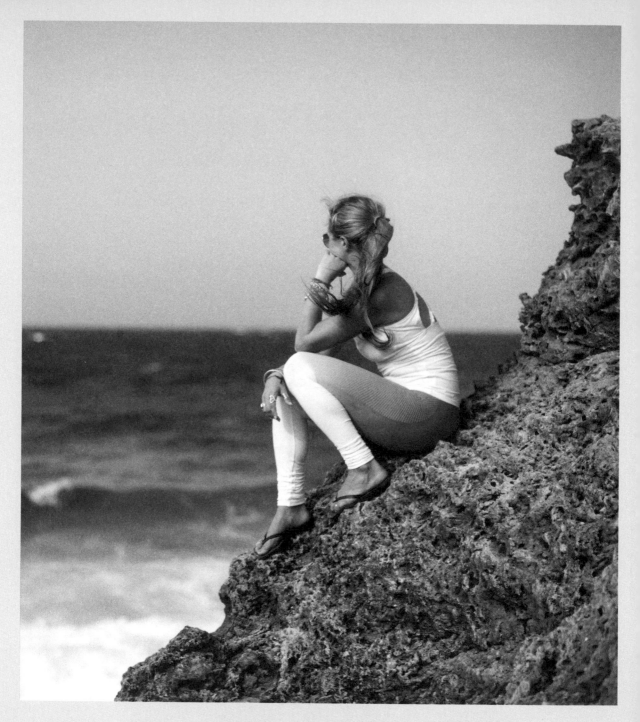

Sit down and close your eyes. You might be sitting in your office chair or your favorite armchair at home. Notice the sounds you hear, the sensations, the smells. Focus on the flow of your breath. Feel your feet on the ground, the chair beneath you, the clothes on your skin, the beating of your heart. Right now, in this moment, reading these words—you are okay. You. Are. Okay.

The only thing that matters is how much you love. In the end it doesn't matter what your body looks like, how successful your career is, how big your house is, how advanced your yoga practice is, or what your bank statement says.

Let me repeat this: *The only thing that matters is how much you love.*

Your purpose on this earth is to love. And love is a two-way street. We give, we get. With love we will turn this crazy world around. With love, we will turn war into peace. Judgment into acceptance. Evil into kindness. You have the ability to change the world, and it all starts with the small acts that make up a day in your life. The key to finding true everlasting happiness lies in this. What you give, you get. To receive love we must first learn how to give it away. To the people closest to us, to our family and friends, and to people we don't know. To acquaintances and people you bump into on the bus. To the people you like and those you don't. To the earth we walk upon and all of the beautiful beings that walk alongside us. And most of all, to ourselves. We must love ourselves in order to receive love from others.

So are you happy to be here? Are you grateful? Or do you feel sadness and regret? You may not feel powerful enough to single-handedly stop a war or world hunger or the injustices that take place around us every day, but you are responsible for your own space and you can change your own vibration. It starts with you, with me, with us as individuals. If every single person directed his or her awareness toward love and trust at this very moment, what would be left to fix? We do not hurt other people if we feel the infinite love present inside us. We are all connected. No matter where you are from, what your beliefs are, or what you look like, we are all in this together.

We all breathe the same air. We are all made up of the same complex combination of molecules. We all share the same big bold beating heart. We've just forgotten it along the way. By giving more love, by becoming compassionate and kind, by forgiving, and by seeing the light in each person, you will start to remember, and from there you *can* single-handedly change the world. You can. You do you, and let me do me. We can only do our best, and when it comes to love, doing our best is always enough.

We are powerful beings. Sometimes we might feel as if we are the victim of our environment, but the fact is, we create the world we live in. The people we encounter on our path are not there by chance, but because we brought them to our life. The experiences we have and the situations we face are here because we each made it so. You are

LOVING INSIGHTS

ॐ The only thing that matters is how much you love.

ॐ Do your best. It will always be enough.

ॐ You are not a victim of your surroundings. You are a powerful being with a choice!

ॐ We must give in order to receive.

ॐ Cultivate mindfulness. Being present in your life and being grateful for what you already have will attract more positive things into your life, and in the end you'll have more and more things to be grateful for. It's a never-ending positive cycle.

ॐ No matter where you are in life, you will always be okay.

ॐ The only thing we can truly know for sure is that things will change. Stay present in what you have and learn to move with the highs and lows of life.

ॐ Allow yourself to feel.

ॐ Love what is. Don't judge. Don't label. Love. Just love.

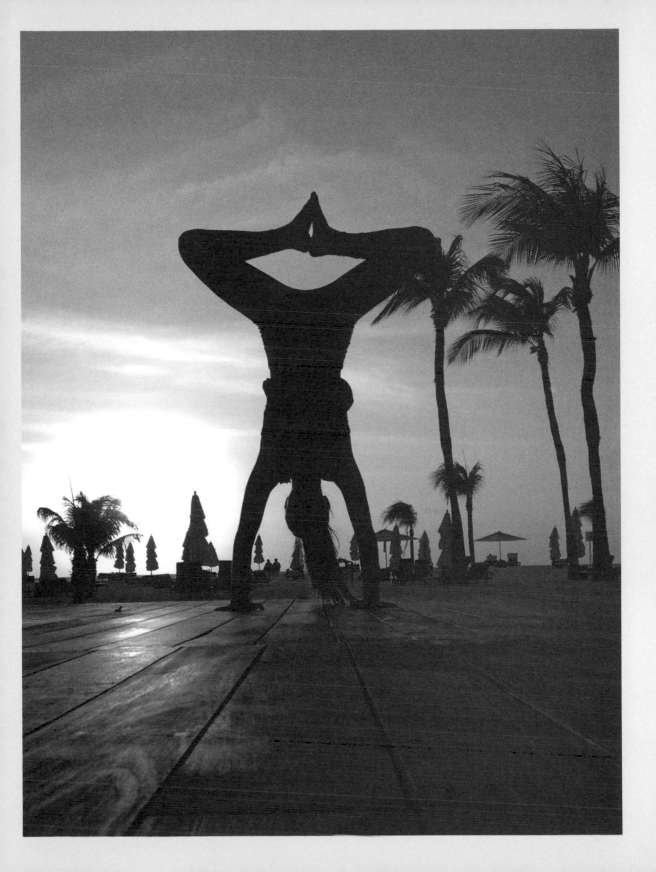

a powerful person with the possibility to manifest anything you like, but most of us do this unconsciously. Depending on what you focus your thoughts and energy on, your situation will change for better or for worse. What does your life look like right now? Are you at peace and content with where you are? Are you manifesting a life of love? Or are you manifesting a life of fear? By becoming aware of our thoughts and realizing the power we have over our situation, we can start to manifest good instead of bad. Focus on what you want to create instead of what you lack. It's very logical: If you think negative thoughts (*I am not good enough/I don't have enough/I am unhappy*), you will have a negative outlook on life and will thus attract more negative experiences into your space. It's a vicious cycle, and we all need to stop it right away.

Begin from where you are. There is beauty all around in this life. Connect to it. Be positive and grateful for the blessings you have. Be here. Don't dwell in the past. Stop thinking in terms of "should have," "could have," or "it would have been better if." You are where you are! You cannot change what was in the past. Why focus on something you cannot possibly do anything about?

What you can do, however, is change your present. It's here, where you are. This is it. Life is now. Change your life by being compassionate, by staying positive, by forgiving, by focusing on love and light and space and gratitude and abundance and happiness. What you direct your energy toward, you attract more of. Meditate on the magical, breathtaking beauty of the world, and soon that magic will be part of your everyday life.

Life is short! What precisely is it that you want to create in your life? Take a moment to write it down. All the things you want for yourself, you must be ready to give to others. If you want love, love. If you want forgiveness, forgive. If you want acceptance, accept. If you want kindness, be kind. It all starts from here. By acting with and sending out love, you will be attuned to the same loving frequency that you need to attract to yourself. It is an absolute truth that we must give in order to receive. And we must know and be clear about what it is we would like our lives to look like.

Our lives tend to get so busy, we spend most of our time simply catching up with what's happening around us, and we forget that we are the creators of our own universe. Life happens for us, not to us. This is something meditation has taught me. By quieting the mind and centering ourselves, we get a chance to step away from the judg-

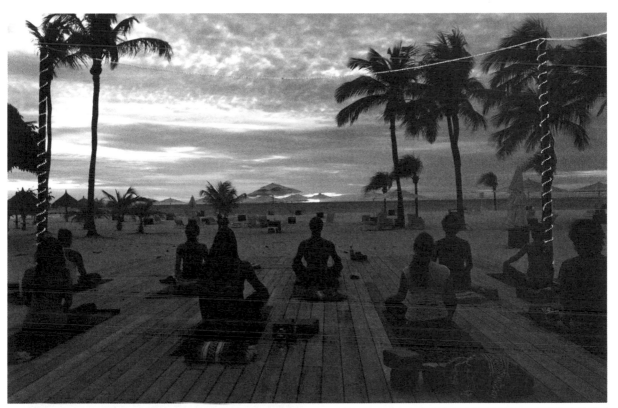

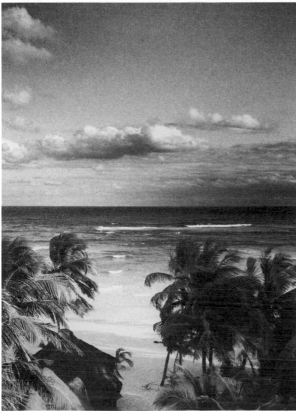

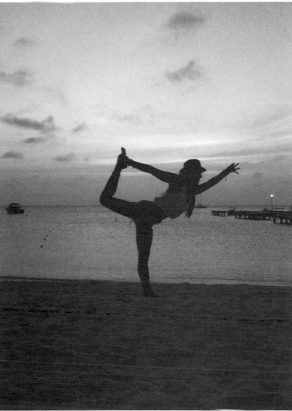

HERBAL TEA

Fresh mint ✺ Fresh sage ✺ Fresh lemon balm

Use a few sprigs of mint, sage, and lemon balm, equal amounts of each. Tear the leaves up so that the aroma is released and put them in a big cup. Add hot water—done!

If you'd rather have iced tea, let it steep for a while and then cool. Add a dash of maple syrup and ice and enjoy on a hot day!

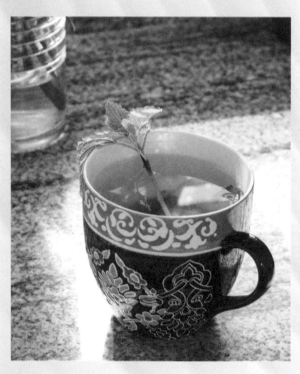

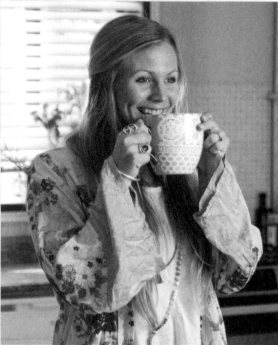

DIRTY HOT CHOCOLATE

1½ cups almond milk ✺ 1 tablespoon maple syrup ✺ 2 tablespoons raw cacao powder ✺ 1 teaspoon maca powder ✺ ½ teaspoon cinnamon ✺ 1 tablespoon instant coffee (optional)

Slowly heat up the almond milk—never let it boil! Pour in the maple syrup. Add all of the dry ingredients and stir well. Drink warm.

Maca contains vitamins B, C, and E. It helps to regulate our hormone levels and can actually stabilize our mood! Perfect for that certain time of the month or when you need a boost.

*"The only thing we know for sure
is that things will always change."*

ments and labels of the mind and move deeper into the truths of our hearts. If we take every single thing our mind tells us seriously, we'll end up neurotic and anxious. The mind tends to be negative and always finds flaws in our present situation. By moving away from the mind we can come back to another universal truth that speaks for us all: *Everything is okay just the way it is.* Even when things are not.

Where are you right now? Focus on what's happening inside yourself right at this moment. Your life is where *you* are. Notice your surroundings. Say you're sitting in your office chair. Notice the sounds you hear, the sensations, the smells. Focus on the flow of your breath. Feel your feet on the ground, the chair beneath you, the clothes on your skin, the beating of your heart.

Right now, in this moment, reading these words, you are okay.

You. Are. Okay. Everything is fine.

It's not until we listen to the fearful thoughts that pass through our minds that we lose the feeling of being cared for. The mind will always tell you something could be better. The mind will focus on all of the worst-case scenarios, thinking this will protect you. But when we don't control what goes on inside of our heads, what we need protection from *is* the mind. Meditate and keep meditating until you have fully embraced this most important truth: *No matter where you are in life, you will always be okay.*

And I'm not just talking about the moments where things are going smoothly, when you're on a high and things are going your way. I'm talking about when they're not. There will be times in your life when you will come to doubt all of these things. Death, disease, divorce, separation, pain—all of these things are inevitable. At some point, whether you like it or not, you will experience most, if not all of them. And I'm not telling you to pretend bad things don't happen, because they do. And they always will. The only thing we know for sure is that things will always change. Nothing is permanent. And when we find ourselves in the middle of trauma, in the middle of crisis, even when you've hit rock bottom and you have no idea how on earth you'll ever find the courage to climb back up, you are still okay. You are okay.

Look around you in that moment, too. What's going on right at that minute? You can still feel your heart beating inside of your chest. Fundamentally, nothing has changed except the story you're telling yourself. Our feelings change like the wind, and when we tell ourselves a story we label good, we tend to be happy. We feel good.

And when we tell ourselves a story we label bad, we tend to be sad. We don't feel good anymore.

You might be sitting in that same office chair and the only thing that has changed is your perception of what has come your way. I'm not saying your pain doesn't matter, because it does. We need pain to teach us what it means to be alive. We need to get the wind knocked out of us so that we can fully appreciate the taste of air. Feel it. Feel it all. But don't ever give up. You are still here. Your heart is still beating. You are okay.

Learn to appreciate the twists and turns of life, and your eyes will open to the magical possibilities of the path you're on. Look around you. It's where you are now, this exact place, that matters. Not where you were yesterday. Not where you'll be tomorrow. It's where you are *now*. And if you happen to find yourself at a particularly bumpy part of the road? Embrace it. Even in darkness, there is light. If things didn't get a little darker once in a while, how would you ever know what the beauty of bright, shining light really means? Without the twists and turns you won't value the smooth ride ahead. Don't judge your life as good or bad. Love what is. And know this—that bumpy road you're on? I'm on it too. We all walk down the same path, and our destination is the same.

You are not alone. ✳

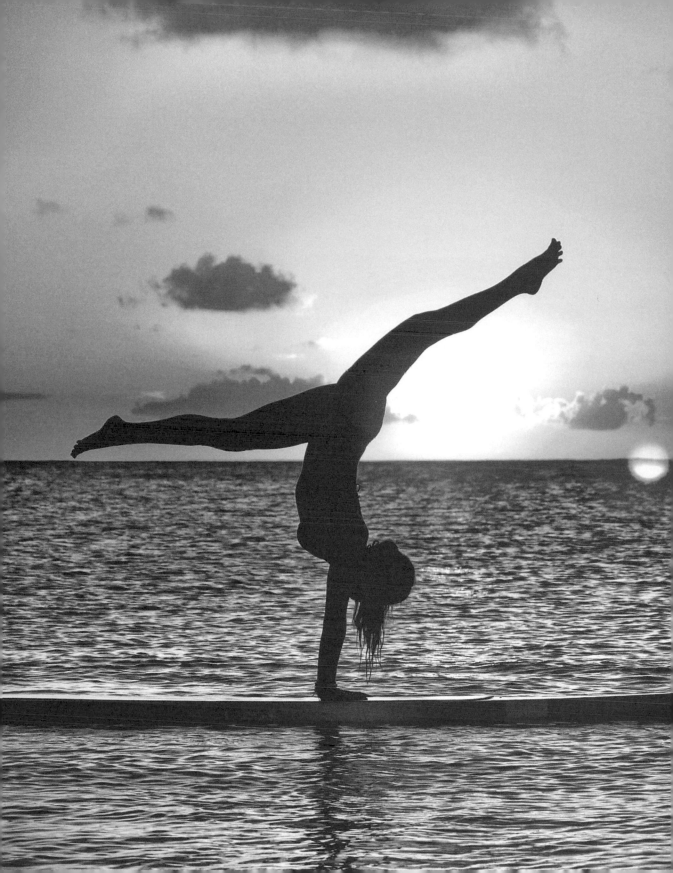

Meditation

Starting up a meditation practice can be more daunting than beginning a physical yoga practice. If you've been practicing yoga for a while you might know that yoga has eight limbs. Asana is one of them, Dhyana (Sanskrit for meditation) is another. Asana, or what we in the Western world call yoga, is created specifically for our busy minds and bodies. By moving together with the breath, by sweating and focusing and working hard to move into different poses, we are forced to stay in the present moment.

While practicing an advanced arm balance, for instance, you won't find it that difficult to stay present in the here and now; you have to, or you'll fall on your face! Meditation—sitting down in stillness, closing your eyes, and spending a few minutes with no company other than yourself—can sound absolutely terrifying because it's so different from the way we live. Our lives are full of sounds and noise and business. We rarely get moments of absolute silence.

In this chapter I'd like to focus on something that's very important in my own yoga practice: meditation. Actually, the physical practice of Asana was invented thousands of years ago as a way to prepare the body for meditation. Have you ever tried sitting in stillness for an entire hour? It's more physically demanding than you might think! If your body is stiff, your hips and lower back will start bothering you fairly quickly.

The physical practice will keep your body soft and spacious enough to sit in stillness without discomfort or distraction.

The yoga pose is not the goal. Becoming flexible is not the goal. Standing on your hands is not the goal. The goal is serenity. Balance. Truly finding peace in your own skin.

The meditation exercise on the next page is anything but daunting. It's simple and requires only five minutes of your time. For meditation, as for yoga, you need to practice. Do you remember how difficult your very first Downward-Facing Dog was? Your first vinyasa? Same thing goes for sitting in silence. In the beginning it's hard, but the more you practice, the easier it will be. A meditation practice can change your life beyond the realm of the body. Meditation helps you create space between you and your circumstances. Meditation inspires calm. Focus. Wisdom. You won't know where your meditation practice is going to take you before you start. The key is to be consistent. Start by meditating for five minutes a day, either right when you wake up or right before you go to bed. After a month of practice, increase your meditation time to ten minutes, then fifteen. Aim to get to twenty minutes of meditation daily. It will make a difference in your life!

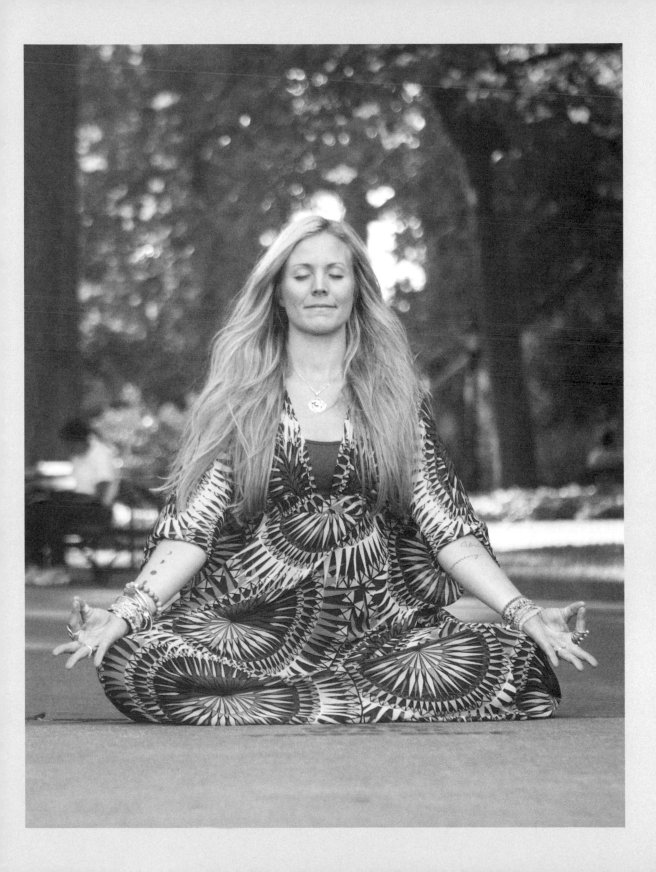

Find a quiet place to sit with no disturbances. Place a small pillow or a folded blanket beneath your sit bones; you will be most comfortable sitting when the creases of your hips are slightly higher than your knees. Set a timer for five minutes; having a set time frame helps your mind settle. Let your hands rest on your knees, palms down. Lengthen your spine and draw the shoulders down your back. Now close your eyes.

Focus on the natural pace of your breath. Notice the gentle expansion and contraction of the low belly. Feel the flow of air through your nostrils and the subtle changes of the body with every breath. Start directing your awareness to the small space you have between the two sides of the breath; the pause between the inhale and the exhale, and the gap between the exhale and the inhale. Stay very, very present with your breath. When thoughts arise, don't judge or resist. Don't try to chase them. Watch your thoughts pass. See if you can, through conscious awareness of the breath, create more space in between each thought. Stay here. Breathe. Be present. When your five minutes are up, bring your hands together at the center of your heart and extend gratitude to everyone and everything you have to be grateful for in life. Repeat to yourself the holiest of all mantras: *thank you, thank you, thank you.* Turn the corners of your mouth into a smile and open your eyes.

Set aside time every day to do this! Gradually increase the time you sit in silence until you're comfortable meditating for twenty minutes each day. Give yourself these moments of peace. Of calm. Of love. Trust that you are on the right path and that life will take you exactly where you need to be. Practice yoga. Meditate. Eat well. Be kind to yourself! Your body, mind, and soul will thank you. ✾

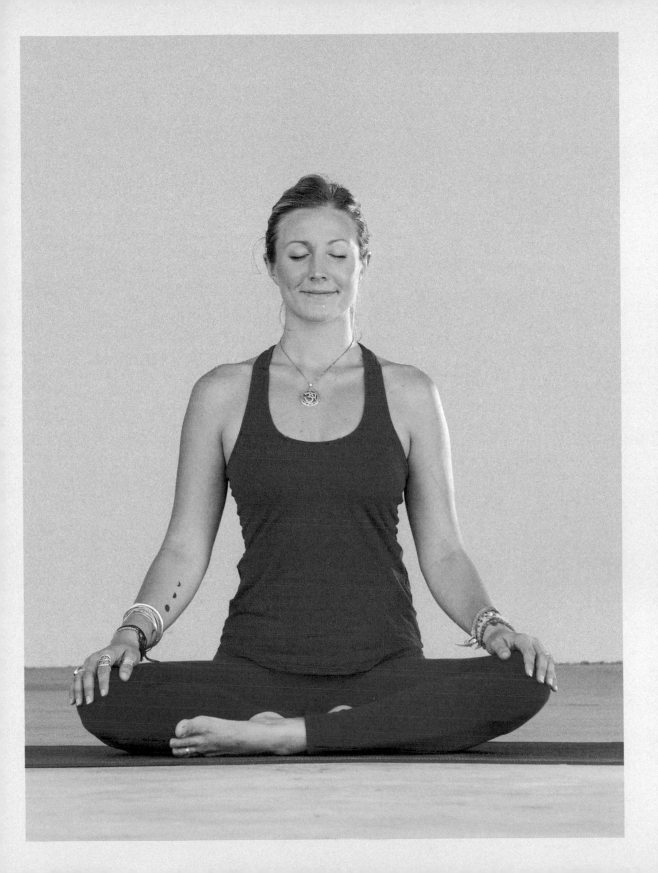

Acknowledgments

This book was written during a year full of high highs and low lows, and if it wasn't for the following people, you wouldn't be holding this beautiful collection of thoughts and inspiration in your hands today! A big thank-you to:

Malin Eklund, Hannah Widell, and Amanda Schulman at Perfect Day Media for believing in me from day one and convincing me to turn the dream of this book into a reality. Thank you to my book agent, Philip Sane, who made sure we ended up in good hands, and to Alexandra Lidén, Åsa Karsberg, and Kai Ristilä from Bonnier Fakta for amazing patience and hard work. Writing a book while traveling is not easy, and countless hours of meetings, e-mails, and phone calls with them, from all corners of the world, resulted in these pages of love. Thank you to my good friend Joyce Husken for giving me a hand with cooking and recipes. A huge thank-you to my friend and teacher Alexis Martin for helping me perfect the yoga section of the book, and to Ben Kane for our beautiful photos.

I want to thank my parents for giving me the courage to go my own way and for always believing in my dreams no matter how crazy they might have seemed. Thank you to my teachers and students for everything you do for me every day and to my followers all across the globe for continuously inspiring me to do my very best.

Last but never least, thank you, Dennis, for everything you do each day. For pushing me to continue writing even when I was lacking inspiration, for creating space for me to work in peace, for taking care of everything that needed to be taken care of so that I could write without distractions. I wrote this book mainly in our kitchen at home in Aruba, at airports all over the world, during yoga retreats, in Brazil, in the United States, and even a little bit during our honeymoon in Greece. If it wasn't for your patience and calm, none of this would have been possible.

And thank you, Pepper, for keeping my feet warm when I was sitting at the computer at home and for making me pause for walks and cuddles just as often as needed.

We miss you. ❀

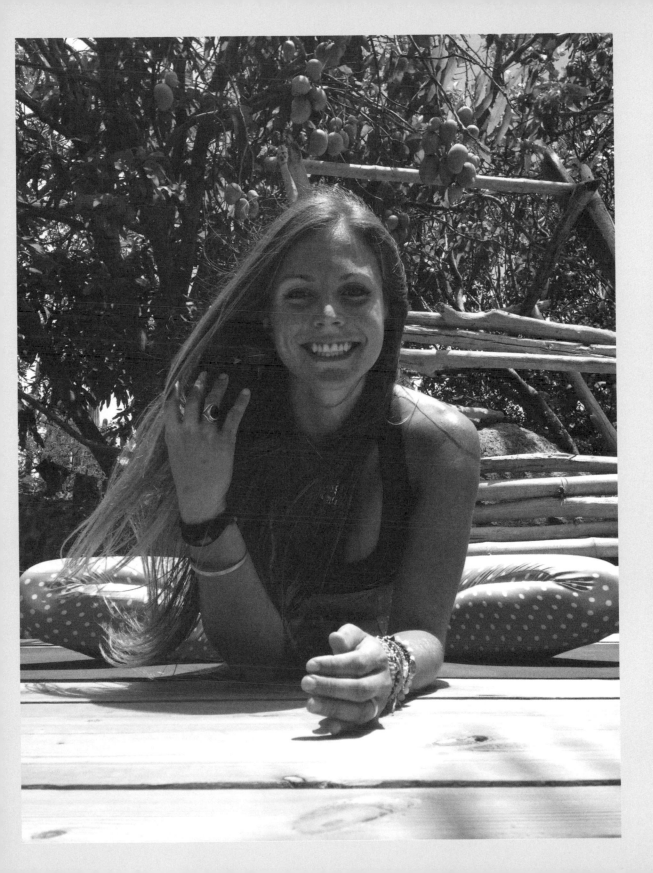

Index

YOGA SEQUENCING

Adho Mukha Vrksasana, 136–37
Agnistambhasana, 45
Ardha Matsyendrasana, 44
Ardha Navasana, 65

Bakasana, 139
Balasana, 99
Big Toe Pose, Reclining, 42
Boat Pose, 65
Bridge Pose, 96, 97
Butterfly, 117

Camatkarasana, 96
Camel Pose, 97
Chaturanga Dandasana, 17, 94
Child's Pose, 99
Cobra Pose, 95
core exercise, eagle variation, 66
Corpse Pose, 34
Crow Pose, 139

Dog, Downward-Facing, 17, 94, 95, 96,
    136, 138
Dog, Upward-Facing, 17, 95
Double Pigeon Pose, 45
Downward-Facing Dog, 17, 94, 95, 96,
    136, 138

Eagle Pose, seated, 68
Eagle Pose, variation, 66
Eka Pada Galavasana, 135
Extended Big Toe Pose, 72–73
Eye of the Needle, 43

Forearm Stand, 134
Flying Pigeon Pose, 135

Garudasana, seated, 68
Gomukhasana Arms, 69

Half Boat Pose, 65
Handstand, 136–37

Handstand against the wall, 138
heart opener, supported, 98
Headstand, 132–33
hip opener, 117

Legs, 90-Degree, 114
Legs-up-the-Wall Pose, 116
leg lifts, reclining, 64
leg stretch, reclining, 42

Navasana, 65
neck stretch, seated, 67

Open Legs, 116

Pigeon Pose, Double, 45
Pigeon Pose, Seated, 114
Pigeon Pose, Flying, 135
Pincha Mayurasana, 134
Plank Pose, 17, 94

Salamba Sirsasana, 132–33
Savasana, 34
Setu Bandha Sarvangasana, 96
shoulder stretch, seated, 68
spinal twist, supine, 43
spinal twist, seated, 44
Sukhasana, 45
Sun Salutation A, 16–18
Sucirandhrasana, 43
Supta Matsyendrasana, 43
Supta Padangusthasana, 42
Surya Namaskar A, 16–18

Tree Pose, 70–71

Upward-Facing Dog, 17, 95
Urdhva Dhanurasana, 97
Ustrasana, 97
Utthita Hasta Padangusthasana,
    72–73

Vinyasa, 94–95
Vinyasa for beginners, 94–95

Viparita Karani, 116
Vrksasana, 70–71

Wheel Pose, 97
Wild Thing, 96

RECIPES

Avocado Soup, Raw, 39

Banana Ice Cream, Raw, 88
Big Green Smoothie, 11

Carrot and Ginger Soup, 110
Chocolate Shake, Yoga-Girl Style, 128

Dirty Hot Chocolate, 148

Green Juice, 11
Granola, Upside-Down in a Jar, 128
Guacamole, 61

Heavenly Hummus, 61
Herbal Tea, 148
Hot Chocolate, Dirty, 148
Hummus, Heavenly, 61

Ice Cream, Raw Banana, 88

Raw Avocado Soup, 39
Raw Banana Ice Cream, 88
Raw Vegan Bounty Bliss, 88

Salad, Superfood, 39
Shake, Chocolate, Yoga-Girl Style, 128
Smoothie, Big Green, 11
Soup, Carrot and Ginger, 110
Soup, Raw Avocado, 39
Superfood Salad, 39

Tea, Herbal, 148

Upside-Down Granola in a Jar, 128

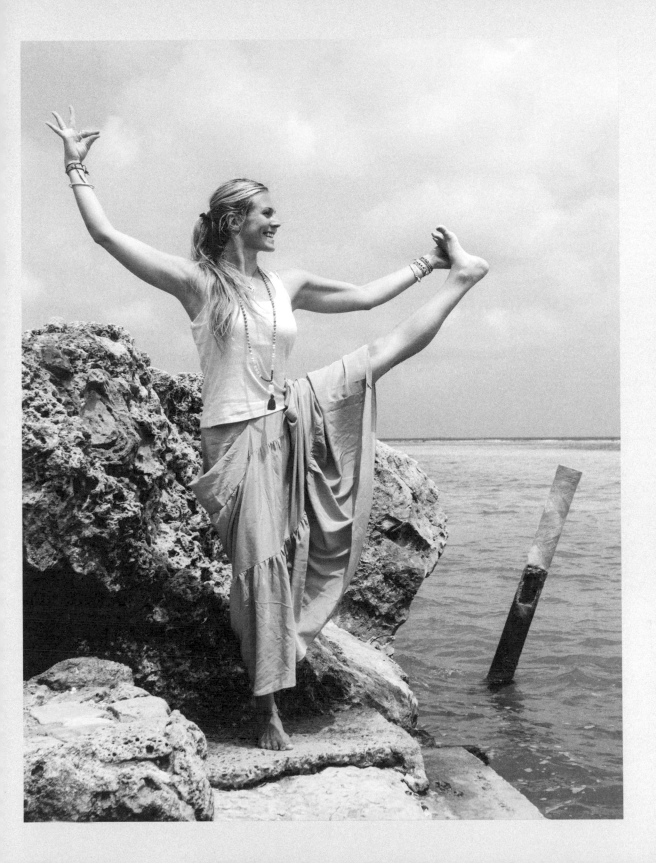

About the Author

Rachel Brathen is a world-renowned yoga instructor who teaches workshops, leads yoga retreats, and gives lectures around the globe.

A native of Sweden, she has been practicing yoga since she was a young teen. After graduating from school she traveled to Costa Rica, and it was there that she found the joy of incorporating yoga into her everyday life. Rachel is known for her free-spirited classes, as well as for sharing pieces of her life, advice, and daily inspiration with her online community of more than one million followers. She currently resides in Aruba with her husband and dogs.

Find her on Instagram @yoga_girl—one of the largest yoga accounts in the world.

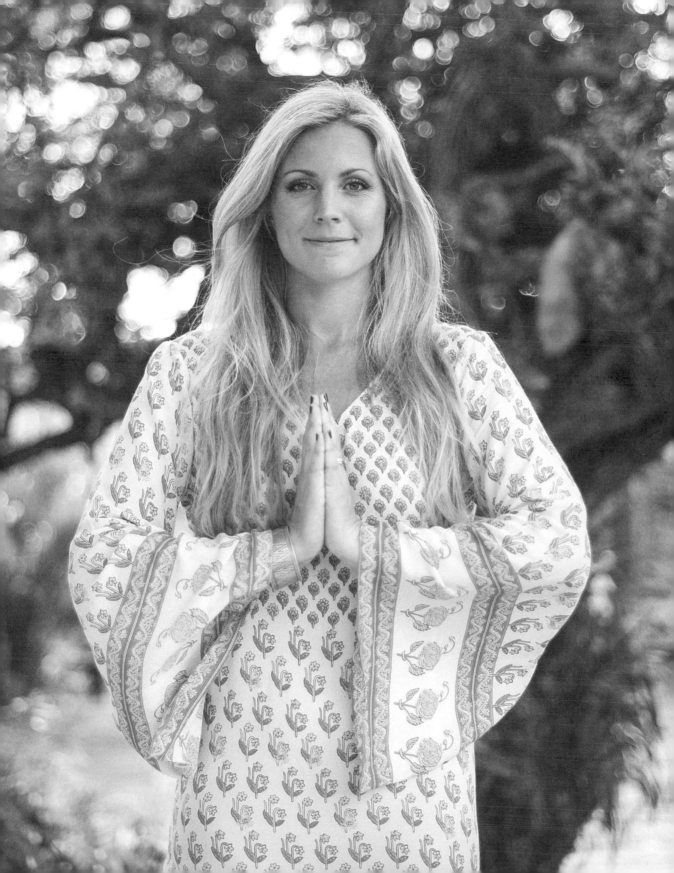

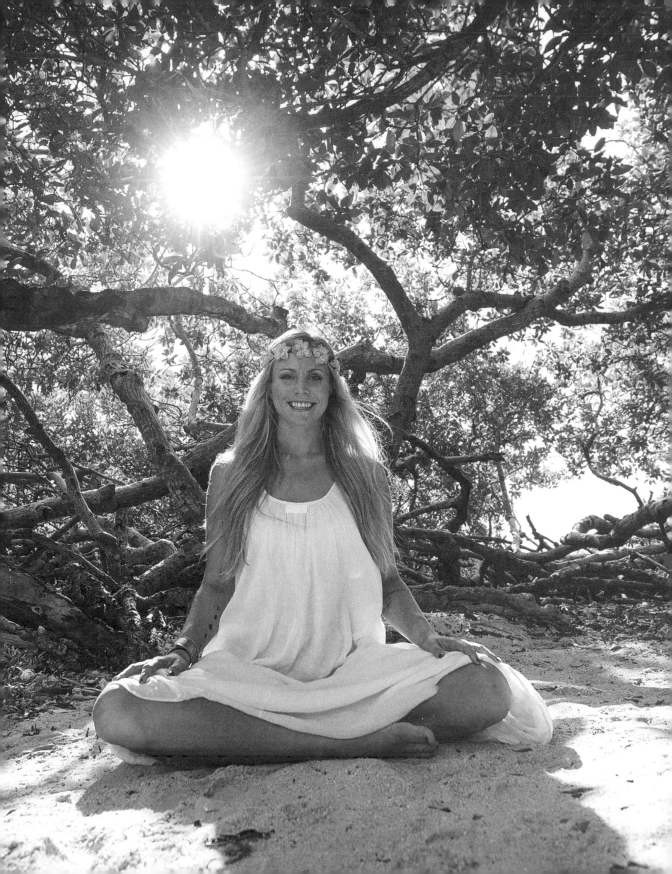

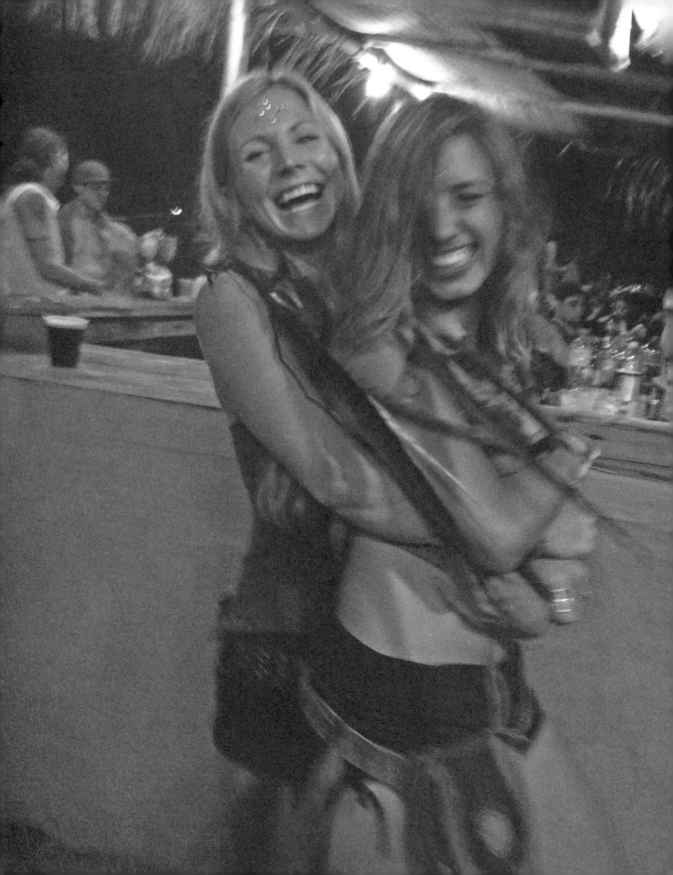

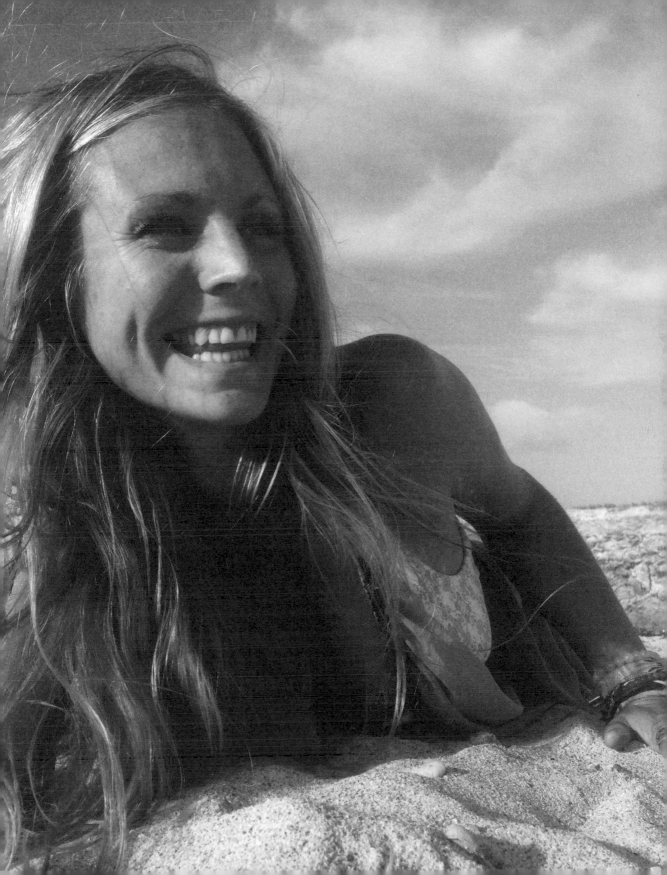

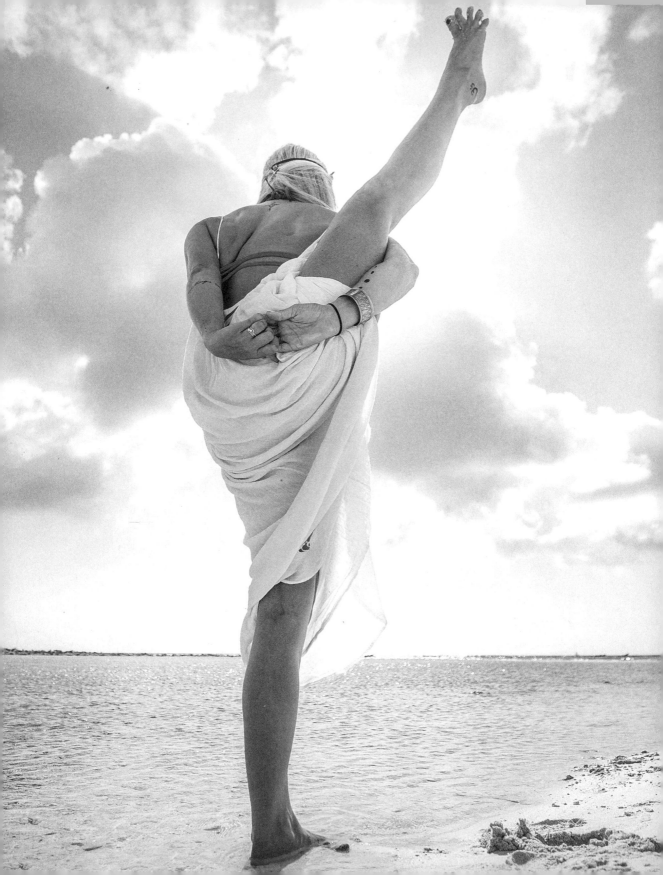